# Malthus, Darwin, Durkheim, Marx, Weber, Ibn Khaldûn:
## On Human Species Survival

# Malthus, Darwin, Durkheim, Marx, Weber, Ibn Khaldûn:
## On Human Species Survival

by

Walter L. Wallace

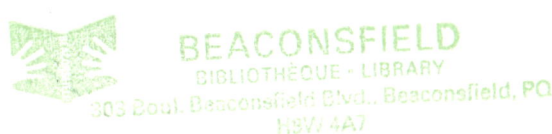

## Gordian Knot Books
*An Imprint of Richard Altschuler & Associates, Inc.*
New York

Malthus, Darwin, Durkheim, Marx, Weber, Ibn Khaldûn: On Human Species Survival. © 2009 by Walter L. Wallace.

For information contact the publisher, Richard Altschuler & Associates, Inc., at 100 West 57th Street, New York, NY 10019, RAltschuler@rcn.com or (212) 397-7233.

Library of Congress Control Number: 2008943120
CIP data for this book are available from the Library of Congress

ISBN: 978-1-884092-78-7
Gordian Knot Books is an imprint of Richard Altschuler & Associates, Inc.

All rights reserved. No part of this publication may be reproduced, stored in a retrieval system, or transmitted, in any form or by any means, electronic, mechanical, photocopying, recording, or otherwise, without the prior written permission of Richard Altschuler & Associates, Inc.

Cover Design: Walter L. Wallace

Cover Layout: Josh Garfield

Figures: Joyce Shih

Printed in the United States of America

To Sarane,

to Jeffrey, Robin, and Aslynn,

and to Sunanda and Anthony

Thought has as its aim . . . the construction of a future reality.
—Émile Durkheim (1960 [1914], 428)

My thanks to Princeton University for providing me with an office and the other physical equipment needed to write this book; to Paul Benaceraff for recommending Bas C. Van Fraassen's book; to Joseph Wisnovsky for recommending Alex Vilenkin's book; to Martin Morand for reading an early draft of chapter 3; and to Charles Westoff for urging me to take another look at Malthus's work.

# Contents

List of Figures     ix

## Part I

1. Introduction: Malthus's and Darwin's Precursor Theories     1

2. Durkheim's Core Sociological Theory: Sociocultural Self-Maintenance     25

## Part II

3. Marx's Supplementary Theory: The Individual Human's Physical (and Psychical) Behaviors     69

4. Weber's Supplementary Theory: The Individual Human's Psychical (and Physical) Behaviors     97

5. The Supplemental Theories of Ibn Khaldûn and Others: Geography and Technology     137

## Part III

6. Summary and Conclusion     161

Appendix: Three Disagreements about Durkheim's Theory     177

Notes     187

References     219

More Detailed Table of Contents     241

Name Index     245

# Figures

| | |
|---|---|
| 1.1. Human Society as a Participant-Throughput System | 19 |
| 2.1. Durkheim's *The Division of Labor in Society* | 38 |
| 2.2. Durkheim's *Suicide* | 47 |
| 2.3. Durkheim's *The Elementary Forms of the Religious Life* | 57 |
| 2.4. Durkheim's *Moral Education* | 64 |
| 3.1. Marx's Pre-Class Division of Labor Labor-Process | 78 |
| 3.2. Marx's Class Division of Labor Labor-Process | 88 |
| 3.3. Marx's Post-Class Division of Labor Labor-Process | 95 |
| 4.1. Weber's Eight Types of Rationality for Comparing "Means," Plus Two Types of "Ethics" for Choosing among "Means" or among "Ends" | 114 |
| 6.1. Constants Proposed by Ibn Khaldûn and Weber, and Variable Mechanisms Proposed by Malthus, Darwin, Durkheim, and Marx, for Human Societal (and Species) Survival | 169 |

# PART I

## Chapter 1

## INTRODUCTION:
## MALTHUS'S AND DARWIN'S PRECURSOR THEORIES

### *Goal of This Book*

The conventional way of understanding and using classical sociological theory claims that knowledge of the political, economic, and other circumstances in which the theories were written and of the persons who wrote them are indispensable. We are told that "a correct appraisal of a particular thought is often difficult, if not impossible, if the social context in which it took root cannot be understood." For example, "you cannot understand [Max] Weber's thought if you fail to place yourself, through an imaginative leap, in the intellectual and social climate in which he wrote" (Coser 1977, xiii, xv). Twenty years later we can still read that "Brief biographies of the classical theorists" (Craib 1997, xv) are essential to understanding the theories they wrote.

This book rejects all such positions. We argue that for comprehending and making empirically descriptive, explanatory, and predictive use of theories, the *only* important thing is the extent to which the theories make empirical sense to readers and users in *their* times and places, not to the *authors* in theirs. We should therefore expect the "correct appraisal" of the theories to change, perhaps radically, with new times, new places, new readers. (Case in point: the twenty-first-century revival of interest in Einstein's "cosmological constant," which we are told he himself thought was the biggest mistake of his life.)

We argue that it simply does not matter who wrote the theories in question—we could just as well give numbers or Greek letters to the theories as name them. It does not matter when or where the writers lived, who they hung out with or fought with, what their genders, ages, socioeconomic statuses, ethnicities, races, or nationalities were, or anything of the sort.[1] After all, who in their right mind would prepare for a trip through unfamiliar territory *not* by perusing an up-to-date roadmap, *not* by getting the car checked out, *not* by filling the gas tank, and so forth, but by reading up on the life and times of the people who invented the gasoline engine, the accelerator, the brake, the steering wheel?

It will surely be noticed, however, that all but one of the classical theories examined here were based on observations made mainly on just a few Western European societies (France, England, Germany, the United States). Only Abdurahman Muhammad Ibn Khaldûn, a Tunisian, wrote about Near Eastern societies, and nothing is said by him or any other theorist here about China, the oldest and the fourth largest of existing civilizations. Nevertheless, the theories discussed here are among the classical Western foundations of all the social sciences and we are concerned with them here because they seem sure to figure into the *global* theory of human sociocultural phenomena as it emerges.

## *The Future of Human Species Survival*

In that global theory we expect that the ongoing *forecasting* of, and planned *preparation* for, likely future threats to the continued survival of the human species will be one of its leading research problems—as it will be of all the empirical sciences. We must admit, however, that *not a single one* of the theories discussed in this book (or to our knowledge in the rest of classical Western sociological theory as well) explicitly mentions concern for the continued survival of the human species. Such survival was just not a problem for classical sociological theory; they took it for granted.

Actually, Charles Darwin does nearly mention human species *extinction* (if not survival) when he tells us that "not one living species will transmit its unaltered likeness to a distant futurity" (1968, 459)—but he stops short of telling us that this eventuality applies to our own species as well as all others. Ibn Khaldûn, too, makes his own near-mention of human species extinction when he says "the great question is now at issue whether man shall henceforth start forwards with accelerated velocity towards illimitable, and hitherto unconceived improvement; or be condemned to a perpetual oscillation between happiness and misery, and after every effort remain still at an immeasurable distance from the wished-for goal" (1967, 2–3). Ibn Khaldûn needs only have added one other possibility to the endlessly forward motion and the endlessly forward and backward motion that he mentions—namely, simply *stopping*, going *extinct*, but he did not.

In this twenty-first-century book, however, the question we ask is this: given the copious paleontological evidence that extinction has already overtaken all but "perhaps a thousandth of the total [number of species] that has wandered our globe" (Kauffman 2000, 74),[2] and given that extinction is now tracking much of even that remnant thousandth (see Kanter 2008), how can we reasonably and responsibly go on *not* trying to forecast, and *not* preparing to protect our own descendants against early species extinction?[3]

Of course, it may seem only natural to focus on our genotypical anatomical and physiological characteristics (that is, the way each of us is organized *within* ourselves) as the sole means of our species' survival. Darwin himself tells us that "*individuals* having any advantage, however slight, over others, would have the best chance of surviving and of procreating their kind. . . . This preservation of favorable [*individual*] variations and the rejection of injurious variations, I call Natural Selection" (1968, 130–131; all italics throughout this book, unless otherwise indicated, are mine).

Only many pages later does Darwin add the essential social science point that the "*swarm* [of honeybees] which wasted least honey in the secretion of wax, having succeeded best . . . will have had the best chance of succeeding in the struggle for existence" (1968, 256)—even though some members of that successful swarm might not have had much of a chance to succeed as individuals. Which is to say, the way a species' organisms are socioculturally organized *among* themselves can be a major (even *the* major) factor in that species' survival chances over and above the way its individual members are organized anatomically and physiologically *within* themselves.

Perhaps Darwin is following up that crucial implication when he tells us that "an advancement in the standard of *morality* . . . will certainly give an immense advantage to one *tribe* [of humans] over another" (1981, 1, 166)—which, as we shall see in chapter 2, almost explicitly anticipates Émile Durkheim's theory of the division of labor as generating such an "advancement" in morality. It was not Darwin, however, but his younger contemporary, Herbert Spencer, who distinguished what he called "*Super*-organic Evolution . . . as including all those processes and products which imply the *coordinated actions of many individuals*" from *individual*-based evolution (1898, 1:4). Despite this advance of Spencer's theory over Darwin's, it still seems fair to say that they both saw *collective* organization as well as *individual* organization as different means that can serve the same end—namely, species survival (see chapter 6 here on equifinality).

The two means of continued species survival mentioned so far (that is, individual organization and collective organization), however, do not seem to have fostered equally powerful human species survival accomplishments in recent history. By 2020 Homo sapiens is expected to reach a roughly forty-seven-fold increase in its global population size over what it was two thousand years ago (see Ward and Brownlee 2000, 284), but since no genotypical changes in our species' individuals have yet been found that might account for such an increase (but see Biello 2007), there is a strong likelihood that, during the most recent two millennia at least, Homo sapiens has improved its species survival chances more through its collective organization than through its individual organization.

## Adding Ongoing Foresight and Planned Preparation to Unforeseen, After-the-Fact, "Natural Selection"

Max Weber claims that empirical science seeks not only "*theoretical* mastery [that is, understanding] of reality by means of increasingly precise and abstract concepts" but also the "methodical attainment of a definitely given and *practical* end [that is, control] by means of an increasingly precise calculation of adequate means" (1946, 293). To this, Karl Mannheim adds his welcome word that "intellectuals" (we would say, more particularly, empirical scientists of all disciplines) should "play the part of *watchmen* [for our species] in what otherwise would be a pitch-black night" (1955, 160–161). Both Weber and Mannheim, then, imply that *foresight and planned preparation* should eventually come to augment "blind, stupid, unforesightful" natural selection (Campbell 1965, 26–27; see also Voight et al.

2006) and the only slightly less blind "sexual selection" of higher organisms (see Darwin 1968, 136; 1981, 2:398). If that were to happen, it would be the first known instance of a species' knowledgeable self-defense against extinction.

We forecast and prepare defenses against many future eventualities of this general sort every day, of course, as when we predict that collisions are more likely to occur at roadway intersections than elsewhere and then we place traffic signs at those intersections as protections against those collisions. Our proposal here is that social scientists should seriously begin to do the same for future sociocultural threats to our species survival.

There is a view, however, that seems to put into question the possibility of such reliable sociocultural forecasting and preparation on the ground that "nonequilibrium systems [such as sociocultural phenomena] can be thought of as computers carrying out algorithms. For vast classes of such algorithms, no compact, lawlike description of their behavior can be obtained" so that, Kauffman implies, we may only be able to observe and cope reactively with "the succession of actions and states as [or rather, *after*] they unfold"—and not predictively and proactively *before* they unfold (1995, 23, 22; also see 2000, 3, 22, 135–139).

It seems clear, though, that the degree of detail required of a given forecast and preparation has to be factored into its reliability (see Lindley 2007, 146–147). For example, Scarlett could reliably predict that tomorrow will be "another day" because "tomorrow" is such a broad generality that every day must be regarded as like every other day (in that, say, the Sun will rise and set). But no one can reliably predict all the chancy mixes of details in any *specific* tomorrow that compel us to regard every tomorrow as a new day rather than just another repeat of countless yesterdays. Physicists can predict with very high reliability that 50 percent of any sizable sample of carbon-14 will decay into nitrogen-14 over about 5,730 years, but they cannot reliably predict *which particular atoms* in the sample will be parts of the 50 percent that decays and which ones will be part of the other 50 percent.

We also suspect that if some astrophysical speculations are right that the universe itself has limits in time and space (beyond which there may exist other universes, both like and unlike our own universe, endlessly), then everything in our universe, including life, has limits too. We now feel pretty sure, for example, that roughly eight billion years passed after the Big Bang before there was an Earth, and that there were roughly two billion years of Earth's existence before there was any life on Earth. After the emergence of that life, two billion more years passed before the species we call Homo sapiens evolved, and it seems a reasonable guess that many more billions of years may pass after our descendants have given rise to some successor species and then itself gone extinct before this particular universe closes shop.

Ward and Brownlee forecast that "the final outcome [not for the universe but for all Earthly life] may be brought about by external sources such as impacts [from outer space] or a nearby supernova, by internal effects such as atmospheric or biological catastrophe, or . . . by increase in the brightness of the central star" (2000, 32). (As sociologists, we are surprised that Ward and Brownlee include no human sociocultural contributions to "the final outcome." Such contributions do seem possible, however, especially given our species' fixation on developing ever more effective weapons of our species' self-destruction.) "Life *on our planet*," Ward and Brownlee conclude, "will eventually be roasted out of existence" (2000, 32).

We emphasize the phrase "on our planet" in that quotation because we believe it possible that Homo sapiens (if it lasts long enough on Earth) will migrate to some other life-supporting planet circling some astronomically nearby star younger than our Sun and so extend the human species' life-span beyond Earth's life-span.[4] Of course, any such successful migration requires a reliable forecast that the destination-planet will actually support human life and will not itself "be roasted out of existence" shortly after our descendants arrive there.

Forecasting and planned preparation to meet likely future events are not new ideas to humankind. But until very recently in our history we have bet largely on mystical prophecy and supplication for them. Moreover, Matthew advises us to "Take *no thought* for the morrow: for the morrow shall take thought for the things of itself"—which seems the essence of 'muddling through.' Now, however, four hundred years after Galileo (and perhaps two thousand years after Matthew), physical scientists *are* taking thought for "the morrow"—developing forecasts and preparations for changes in climatological, geological, ecological, and astronomical phenomena that can be dangerous to our species—and we believe social scientists should try to do the same for human sociocultural phenomena.

The idea has been around for a long time, however, that if we social scientists could carry out the kind of rigorously controlled and replicable experiments that physicists do, sociologists too might invent reliable techniques of foresight and preparation. But we know there are ethically and practically impassable barriers to even trying such experimentation with human sociocultural phenomena. For example, Campbell says that in a true experiment "one needs optimally to be able to randomly assign persons to [different] experimental treatments and to enforce 100% participation in these treatments. . . . [Also,] the participants should be unaware of the experiment [and] unaware that other people are deliberately being given different treatments" (1958, 14–15). That is an inordinately tall order when the experimental subjects are humans.

So we have a choice: we can either just *forget* about forecasting and preparing for our species' future and stick to taking-things-as-they-come and muddling through, or we can try to find some way of forecasting and preparing *approximately*—not completely or exactly, but well enough at least to identify roads we should *not* take because their probabilities of leading to extinction are prohibitive.

Fortunately, a new, twentieth-century, instrument of the empirical sciences seems to promise that kind of approximation.[5] In what are called "agent-based" computer simulations, the behaviors of multiple individual sociocultural participants are programmed, and their past, present, and likely future interactions are simulated in computer runs. Outputs of such simulations, tested for accuracy against empirical findings of the real world, may then be used as inputs to the next higher level of simulation, and so on hierarchically up toward simulating what we believe is the global human society that has been, and still is (despite much of the daily news), fitfully emerging since the first ethnicity-consolidating empires were formed around five thousand years ago (see Wallace 1997).

Epstein and Axtell, in introducing their now-classic demonstration of an agent-based computer simulation, put the argument for that simulation this way:

> Agents are the "people" of [computer simulated human] societies. Each agent has internal [psychophysical] states and behavioral rules. Some states are fixed for the agent's life, while others change through [physical] interaction with other agents or with the ex-

ternal environment.... [F]undamental social structures [and culture structures]... emerge from the [physical] interaction of [multiple] individuals operating in [technologically] artificial environments under rules that place only bounded demands on each agent's [psychical] information and [psychophysical] computational capacity. We view artificial societies as [sociocultural] laboratories, where we attempt to "grow" certain social structures [and culture structures] in the computer. (1996, 4, italics removed)

A couple of years earlier, Contractor and Siebold pointed out that "artificial [computer-simulated] societies" can be consequential not only for what we have already quoted Weber calling the "practical end[s]" of human sociocultural life but also for achieving what he called "theoretical mastery" of that life. Thus, Contractor and Siebold claim that "although human intellect is capable of articulating nonlinear relationships, it is limited in its capacity to mentally construe the long-term.... The role of computer simulations... is to help us understand ... the implications of our verbal theories and propositions. Without them it is well nigh impossible for us to appreciate the long-term implications [of those theories and propositions]" (1993, 542, 557).

So we have the possibility of doing both some "practical" work of *forecasting* likely future events in human sociocultural phenomena and *preparing for* those events through computer simulations, and we may, at the same time, do some "theoretical" work of *explaining* human sociocultural events, past, present, and potential future.

A further implication relates to Davidsson's warning that "to create a simulation model from a sociological theory stated in a natural language, all assumptions etc. must be described explicitly and formally... [and] every parameter in the simulation model must be given a value" (2002, 4; also see Goldspink 2000). We should add to this statement that when dealing with *multiple* theories, as we sociologists often do, we should first try to integrate that multiplicity into a *single* theory using a single conceptual vocabulary. Indeed, a single basic sociological vocabulary seems already implicit in the classical theories we examine here, and this book will try to demonstrate that claim.

## *Our Analytical Strategies*

We rely on two broad strategies in that demonstration. Strategy A is to divide the theories we examine into three groups. The first group includes two theories that we identify as logical *precursors* of classical sociological theories regarding human sociocultural (and, by implication, species) survival—namely, the theories of Thomas Malthus (1766–1834) and Charles Darwin (1809–1882). The second group of theories contains only Émile Durkheim's (1858–1917) theory because it expresses what we believe is the *core* idea of all sociological theories—namely, that *human societies* are partly *self-maintaining*.[6]

The third group of theories contains theories that *supplement* Durkheim's core idea by pointing to certain biological features of *human* participants that contribute crucially to human sociocultural self-maintenance (although Durkheim's theory relied on at least two such features—namely, the human abilities *physically* to "labor" (and to commit "suicide"), and *psychically* to think "morally"). The theory of Karl Marx (1818–1883) and his collaborator Friedrich Engels (1820–1895) stresses, first, contributions made by genetically evolved *physical* needs and abilities of the individual participants in specifically human societies, and second, the contributions made by those participants' *psychical* abilities to forecast and prepare to meet future exigencies. The theory expounded by Max Weber (1864–1920) reverses the importance of these two abilities—stressing, first, contributions made by genetically evolved *psychical* needs and abilities of those participants, and paying only minor attention to their *physical* needs and abilities. The theory of Ibn Khaldûn (1332–1406) and his more recent intellectual descendants stresses contributions made by the cosmically evolved *geographical* and the socioculturally evolved *technological* external environments of human sociocultural participants.[7]

Strategy B is somewhat more complicated than strategy A in dealing with the theories examined here. Strategy B derives from the writer having earlier identified some generic concepts that seem present in all three groups of theories identified in strategy A above (see Wallace 1983, 1994, 1997)—and that link all these theories together. Here is a brief explication of the concepts we have in mind.

We accept Durkheim's ideas of *social structure* and *culture structure* (although he doesn't call them that) as the chief generic mechanisms of human sociocultural self-maintenance. To see what we mean by these concepts, it may be useful to turn back a couple of pages in this book to the indented quotation from Epstein and Axtell. We inserted bracketed specifications there that distinguish the authors' references to individuals' *physical behaviors* (that is, roughly speaking, their metabolic, sensory, locomotive, and manipulative needs and abilities) from their references to individuals' *psychical behaviors* (that is, again roughly speaking, their cognitive, cathectic, and conative—or existence-belief, emotional affect, and behavior-dispositional—needs and abilities). We also distinguished, in that quotation, between Epstein and Axtell's references to *multiple* individuals' *social structures* (that is, their *collective* physical behaviors) and references to multiple individuals' *culture structures* (their *collective* psychical behaviors).[8]

We claim that the classical theorists discussed here regard these two concepts—social structure, and culture structure—as the primary mechanisms of human sociocultural self-maintenance. The reason for this primacy is left only implicit in Merton's, and in Kroeber and Parsons's, and Parsons's (see note 8), original distinctions between "social structure" and "culture structure" but that reason is the significant degree of causal *independence* between human *action* and human *thought*.

That is, we claim that when we see only a social structure (two or more individuals physically *doing* something together), *we cannot tell from that observation alone what thoughts, emotional feelings, and/or behavior-dispositions those individuals are experiencing.* In short, humans can do the same *physical* things (for example, vote for or against the same candidate, attend or decline to attend the same school or place of worship, work or not work for the same employer, live in the same town, and so on) for quite different *psychical* reasons, and vice-versa.

That degree of causal independence, indeed, seems to be why establishing a legal defendant's psychical *intention* is often an essential factor in determining his or her degree of punishable guilt for having performed some prohibited physical act that is not in question. And what parent has not asked her or his child "What were you *thinking!?*" in exasperation when something unusual their child has done comes to their attention? This independence is also the basis for Merton's distinction in sociocultural structure between "manifest" (culture structurally intended and recognized) and "latent" (unintended and unrecognized) social structural functions (see 1957, 51),[9] and why Weber warns us that "in a given social relationship . . . 'friendship,' 'love,' 'loyalty,' 'fidelity to contracts,' 'patriotism,' on one side may well be faced with *an entirely different attitude* on the other. In such cases the parties associate *different* meanings with their [*similar*] actions" (1978, 27).

In sharp contrast with these views, Durkheim insists that a given social structure is always and everywhere supported by *one and the same* culture structure: "the [culture structural] morality of each people is directly related to the social structure of the people. . . . The connection is so intimate that, given the general character of the morality observed in a given society . . . one can *infer* the nature of that society, the elements of its structure and the way it is organized" (1973a, 87).

We think Weber is right and Durkheim is quite wrong on this point. We argue that different culture structures can be, and often are, associated with the same social structure, and vice-versa—even though certain culture-and-social associations may be more empirically typical than others. The result is that we cannot simply *deduce* one from the other; we have to look and see what is actually the case and build up *empirical estimates* of the probabilities that a given sort of culture structure is associated with a given sort of social structure or vice-versa. Those probabilities may turn out to be quite different from what we expect and may vary from place to place and time to time. Such differences are much of what we mean when we say human history is not mechanical.

Given this primary distinction between the social structure and the culture structure of human societies and other human collectivities, we need at least three further definitions for our discipline: (1) a definition of *sociocultural phenomena* generically speaking, (2) a definition of *societies* as distinguished from other sociocultural phenomena, and (3) a definition of specifically *human* societies.

## Proposed Generic Definitions of Sociocultural Phenomena and Societies, and of Specifically Human Societies

The generic definition of a *sociocultural phenomenon* that we believe underlies all classical sociological (and sociobiological) theories—but none of them explicitly—is simply this: an *interorganism behavior regularity*. This definition tells us that a sociocultural phenomenon is being observed whenever we see, at minimum, that if one individual organism does something—and/or, by our inference, thinks or feels something—at least one other individual organism regularly (not necessarily always or everywhere) does and/or thinks or feels something. The *descriptive* research problem is to detail the "somethings" that are done and/or thought or felt and the interorganism regularity that characterizes those behaviors. The *explanatory* research problem is to find out why this regularity existed or exists; and the *predictive* research problem is to assess the probability that that explanation and its resulting regularity will exist in the future.

Of course, when we are studying culture structure, we have to indicate the observable indicators (such as speech or other physical sign-making) that we take to represent psychical behaviors—the latter not being directly observable to outside observers without special instruments (see Mead 1962, 25, 132–134)—and we must be careful not to take the same indicator for both physical and psychical behaviors. The behavior regularity that constitutes a sociocultural phenomenon can exist in any geographical (more generally, spatial—because humans now engage in extraterrestrial sociocultural phenomena) and temporal location large or small, and in any technological modification of that location. The participating organisms may be many or few, and they may belong to one biological species or many.

Finally, the sociocultural phenomenon in question may be called a dyad, swarm, society, troop, or whatever.

The generic definition of a *society* that we propose here sees it as a *predominantly single-species participant-throughput system*.[10] This means, essentially, that a society (and a species) tends to last much longer than any single generation of its individual participants. In a society, individuals of the appropriate species enter it in various ways (birth, immigration, capture). They become acclimated to the system's behavior regularities by some combination of maturation and socialization and participate in those regularities for a time. Finally, all individual participants leave the system in various ways (death, emigration, capture). Meanwhile, the system is constantly recruiting new participants as replacements for those who leave it.

A *human* society is so-called because its participants belong predominantly to the human biological *species* (though tens of millions of dogs, cats, and other domesticated animals also participate in human societies—along with a large number of food animals and a gigantic number of feeding microorganisms). The one-dominant-species characteristic of a society enables participants of that species to employ the same means of communication (for example, human speech as compared to honeybee waggle dance), and to organize production, distribution, and consumption of the same geographical resources and the same means of defense against outside enemies.

In defining a society as a *participant-throughput system*, we propose an analogy with the way a wave of water moves across a lake, say, separately or with other roughly similar waves—that is, through the wave's continuous constituent-*intaking*, constituent-*organizing*, and constituent-*outletting* processes. The constituents in question (water molecules) are taken into the wave, have their behaviors changed to conform, more or less, with the established behaviors of their immediate predecessors, and every constituent may (and finally must) leave the wave through its outletting processes.

In human societies, the behaviors of newly in-taken participants are changed as they mature to conform to older participants' behaviors in three types of "institutions," which we shall call participant-intaking (e.g., families, immigration agencies, schools), participant-organizing (see below), and participant-outletting (e.g., emigration, imprisonment, hospitalization, funerary agencies). All participants have active and inactive roles in all three types of institutions and each or the latter is made up of organizations which are, in turn, composed of participant behaviors functionally appropriate to them. In this book we concentrate on our theorists' images of the particular kinds of participant-*organizing* organizations into which in-taken and acclimatized human participants are allocated. These images seem to fall into the following four types:

• *Economic* organizations collect, manufacture, distribute, and consume *wealth*—that is, physical materials and energy harvested from the geographical environment, variously reconstructed (for example, into means of subsistence—including oxygen, water, food, shelter, rest, recreation, and medication—for individual participants and for technological instruments that produce and distribute such subsistence).

• *Political* organizations accumulate, administer, and enforce (with legitimized police and military organizations) decision-making *power* in control of participant interrelations with each other and with participants in other societies.

• *Religious* organizations produce and distribute to participants various degrees of psychical *honor* (prestige, charisma, blessedness) and *self-confidence* ("Omnipotent gods are our allies, so our enemies had best surrender before it is too late!").[11]

- *Informational* (educational-scientific-legalistic-journalistic) organizations produce, combine, and distribute empirical *knowledge* and practical *know-how* of the world which is used by participants to achieve adaptations to, and control over, that world, increasingly including the society itself.[12]

These four types of organizations within the human societal participant-*organizing* institution and their general causal interrelations are diagrammed in figure 1.1, together with more summary representations of the participant-inletting and participant-outletting institutions. Note that this figure also implies general relationships among current sociological specialties—namely, those studying natality, immigration, and schooling (participant-intaking) organizations in human societies, those studying mortality, emigration, and imprisonment (participant-outletting) organizations in those societies, and those studying economic, political, religious, and informational participant-organizing organizations there. This book, by the way, contains several schematic diagrams of this sort; they are meant to summarize the principal structures and causal relations on which our verbal discussions rest and which they elaborate.

The rest of this chapter examines the theories of Malthus and of Darwin, using the vocabulary introduced above, as two logical precursors of Durkheim's core sociological theory.

## *Malthus's and Darwin's Precursor Theories*

Malthus tells us that "The principles on which [his theory depends] have been explained in part by Hume, and more at large by Dr. Adam Smith." Those principles include, Malthus says, the proposition that "First . . . *food* is necessary to the existence

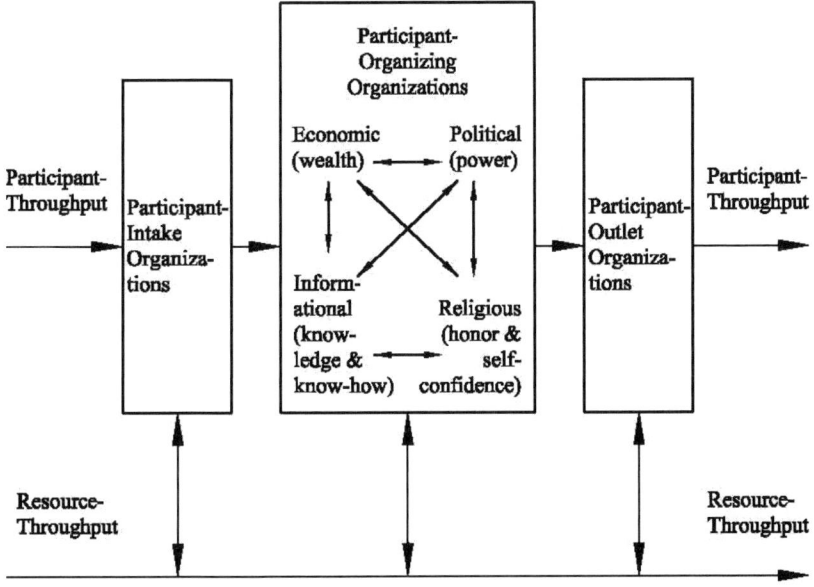

Figure 1.1. Human Society as a Participant-Throughput System

of man [and second] the *passion between the sexes* is necessary [to the species' reproductive intaking], and will remain nearly in its present state" (1966, 8, 11). Malthus then hypothesizes what he regards as the fixed relative powers of these two variables: "the power of [human] population [to reproduce itself] is *indefinitely greater* than the power in the earth to produce subsistence for man." From this claim Malthus draws the practical species-survival conclusion that "the effect of these two unequal powers [i.e., subsistence-production and biological reproduction] *must be kept equal*" by restraining the growth of population (1966, 13–14).[13]

Then, although Malthus says he believes that the unequal powers of reproduction and subsistence are divinely determined (see 1966, 346, 361–393), he recommends not religious activity but secular political activities to keep those powers equal—namely, "preventive checks" to restrain future population growth, and "positive checks" to cut back present population size (see 1966, 62, 63, 71, 99–100, 139).[14]

Malthus forecasts, however, that such "checks" cannot be applied "without producing misery or vice" among the persons to whom they are applied. For example, although war is clearly an effective "positive" check on a society's population, "war is vice," Malthus says, "and the effect of it, misery; and none can doubt the misery of want of food" (1966, 37, 52). Such negative side-effects, however, are the price to be paid for holding back humankind's intrinsic tendency to slide into extinction through unsustainable participant-intake. That price, Malthus says, "form[s] the great difficulty that to me appears insurmountable in the way to the perfectibility of society" (1966, 16).

Malthus adds to this forecast two others—namely, (1) that "in every society that has advanced beyond the savage state, a class of proprietors and a class of laborers *must necessarily exist*" (1966, 287–288; see also 207), and (2) that it is unlikely "that the lower classes of people in any country, should ever be sufficiently free from want and labor to attain any high degree of intellectual improvement" (1966, 217–218; see also Veblen 1979, 204). Although he claims that "the present great inequality of property . . . must certainly be considered as an evil, and every institution that promotes it is essentially bad and impolitic" (1966, 287), it is the *size* of that inequality, not its mere existence, that Malthus finds objectionable. Therefore, he favors its *moderation*, not its elimination: "It is probable, that too great, or too little excitement, [either] extreme poverty, or too great riches, may be alike unfavorable . . . to the growth of mind," so that "if we could find a mode of government, by which, the numbers in the extreme regions would be lessened, and the numbers in the middle regions increased, it would be undoubtedly our duty to adopt it." However, Malthus cautions, "the extreme parts could not be diminished beyond a certain degree . . . [for if] no man could hope to rise, or fear to fall, in society . . . the middle parts would not certainly be what they now are" (1966, 367–369). Merton refers to this as "relative deprivation," implying, but not discussing, its opposite, relative satisfaction (1957, 227–236).[15]

One imagines that Marx, if he read the *moderationist* views just quoted from Malthus (and he could well have done so; he cites Malthus frequently, at 1967, 1:162, 213, 313, 352, 507, 529, 557, etc.), may have been inspired to advance his own markedly *extremist* claim that "in present capitalist society the material etc. conditions have at last been created which enable and compel the workers to *lift* [that is, to *eliminate*] this social curse [of class inequality]" (1969, 3:14–15) by abolishing the entire human class division of labor—top to bottom—and substituting for it a new automatic subsistence-producing technology that would be directed by finally classless human beings (see chapter 3).

Malthus may also have provided Darwin with a point of departure for the latter's theory by declaring that he (Malthus) had "*taken no notice of emigration* for obvious reasons" (1966, 208, but see 24, 52). (Darwin cites Malthus's work [1968, 33, 68, 117; 1981, 1:131, 132, 134]; see also Keynes [1983, 359–364]; Jewell [1983, 365] so we know that Darwin, as well as Marx, read Malthus.) The "obvious reasons" in question, Malthus says, lie in the attitudes of migrants as well as in the societies receiving them: "We well know . . . how much misery and hardship men will undergo in their own country, before they can determine to desert it" (1966, 208–209, but see 24).

Darwin, however, seizes on this very factor of which Malthus says he took "no notice," namely, *migration*—that is, participant-outlet in one societal location and participant-intake in another—as a process that can long forestall the extinction of all populations. In Darwin's words, "all the grand leading facts of geographical distribution [of life forms] are explicable on the theory of *migration* . . . together with subsequent modification and the *multiplication of new forms*" (1968, 393)—that is, *speciation.*

Accordingly, instead of *dying* out (or never having been born), Darwin says the excess members of a population may *migrate* out into some new Earthly location where they find more subsistence and less competition (see 1968, 117, 128–129, 229; cf. 224). Across many generations thereafter, the now separate migrant and nonmigrant parts of the original population of living organisms would diverge genotypically and eventually become distinct, noninterbreeding, biological species. That original population will thereby have succeeded in populating more of Earth's livable habitats with more of its descendants than it could have had it remained undivided.

In a word, then, biological *evolution*—that is, the sequence of *competition* at home, *migration* out of that competition by some losing competitors, and the latter's *speciation* into a new population comprising, perhaps, a new society from which a new migration may then spring—is Darwin's *self-maintaining mechanism for life itself.*

While Malthus, then, proposes restraints on a human society's participant-intaking that can at best achieve only a temporary *stalemate* with extinction, Darwin proposes a process that can, through differentiation, make long-term *gains* in the total global population of living things (see Diamond 1999, 218; Dawkins 1987, 267; Leakey and Lewin 1992, 57, 85, 213). Indeed, the result of Darwin's process, so far, is that from the single species in which Earthly life seems to have originated some 3.7 billion years ago,[16] by now there have evolved, Kauffman says, "some hundred million species" (2000, 74)—which, as we have already seen, he estimates represents only a thousandth of the total number that have existed—while Ward and Brownlee assert that "the world has [now] attained the highest level of biological diversity ever in its history" (2000, 284).

Specifically regarding the human participant-intake and participant-outlet (migratory) processes of recent centuries, Cohen tells us that "since 1600, the human population increased from about half a billion to nearly six billion. . . . Within the lifetime of some people now alive, world population has tripled"—but, Cohen says, "the possibility must be considered seriously that the number of people on the Earth has reached, or will reach within half a century, the *maximum* number the Earth can support in modes of life that we and our children and their children will choose to want" (1995, 367–368). However, "we and our children and their children" may conceivably "choose to want" only a very large population combined with a very high mode of life—thereby threatening our species with the extinction that Malthus almost forecast.

Should "we and our children," then, restrain global human society's population size as Malthus implies? Or should our species plan to migrate to another planet and speciate there as Darwin says? Or should we simply sit tight and eventually go extinct as so many other species have done?

\*

The next chapter focuses on what we regard as Durkheim's core sociological theory. This theory modifies Darwin's migration-

and-speciation (i.e., differentiation) mechanism of species life-survival, as Darwin's theory modifies Malthus's no-migration-but-population-restraint mechanism.

## Chapter 2

## DURKHEIM'S CORE SOCIOLOGICAL THEORY: SOCIOCULTURAL SELF-MAINTENANCE

We begin this chapter by taking up some of Émile Durkheim's general comments about sociology and human sociocultural phenomena because they set the stage for considering four of his works and their joint relation to the central issue of this book—namely, human species survival.

Durkheim tells us that sociology "can be justified only if there are realities which deserve to be called social *and which are not simply aspects of another order of things*" (1960c, 363; see also 1982a, 162; Peyre 1960, 24). But almost a hundred years after his death, one can wonder whether, while Durkheim was alive, breathing, eating, drinking, walking around in sunlight every day, looking up at the stars every clear night, he could really have believed that "social realities" were *cut off from everything else in the universe* and therefore "*not* simply aspects of another order of things."

A few years earlier than Durkheim, however, Auguste Comte had implied the very same cutting-off of sociocultural phenomena by claiming that "no *social fact* can have any scientific meaning till it is connected with some *other social fact*" (1896, 2:245). Despite Durkheim's detailed critique of many other aspects of Comte's theory, Durkheim did not acknowledge Comte's priority in this view (but see 1982b, 194–195) but went on repeatedly to assert, on his own, that "it is in the nature of society itself that we must seek the explanation of social life"; that "the determining cause of a social fact must be sought among antecedent social facts"; "the function of a social fact must always be sought in the relationship that it bears to some social end"; "the primary origin of social processes of any importance must be sought in the constitution of the inner social environment"; "a social fact cannot be explained except by another social fact"; "sociology is . . . itself a distinct and autonomous science"; "society is a reality *sui generis*" (1982a, 128, 134, 135, 162; 1974, 29; 1979, 35; 1994, 19; 1995, 15), and the startling clincher that we are *"prohibited from assimilating [social facts] . . . into the general properties of organized matter"* (1982a, 162, 163). Judging from those claims, then, and contrary to everything else we now think we know about the world as humans experience it, Durkheim did indeed argue that "social realities" should be regarded as completely cut off from everything else in the world.[1]

Nevertheless, it is exactly this *sociocultural self-maintenance* idea of Durkheim's (and Comte's) that is our ground for identifying his theory as the *core* of all sociological theories—although both theorists exaggerated the point. Nowadays, it is thought that almost everything now known to empirical science (the possible exception, this nonspecialist supposes, may be subatomic "virtual particles") is part of 'the great chain of being' and is thereby partly self-maintaining—so ruling out detailed divine causation of each and every phenomenon each moment of its existence.

Once we accept the principle of the collective self-maintenance of phenomena as every empirical science's most fundamental working hypothesis, the next question is *how and to what degree do various kinds of phenomena accomplish their self-maintenance* and how do *other* phenomena contribute to those phenomena's self-maintenance?

Now besides all the quotations just made, Durkheim also tells us that "societies are made up of a number of *parts* added on to each other," and that "since the nature of any composite necessarily depends upon the nature and the number of the *elements* that go to make it up and the way in which these are combined, these characteristics are plainly those which we must take as our basis" (1982a, 111). But then Durkheim strives hard to avoid acknowledging *individual human organisms* as elements of societies. "The constituent parts of every society," he says, "are themselves *societies* of a simpler kind. A people is produced by the combination of two or more peoples that have preceded it. If therefore we knew the simplest society that ever existed . . . we should only have to follow the way in which these simple societies joined together and how these new composites also combined" (1982a, 112; see also Spencer 1898, 467). Thus, Durkheim determinedly looks the other way when *human individuals* come up as constituting constitutive elements of both the "societies of a simpler kind" that he mentions and the more complex societies that derive from compounding simpler ones.

We are not arguing, of course, that Durkheim was *unaware* that individual organisms are present in all societies.[2] We are arguing that he implied, first, that those individuals may be discounted as being only passive conduits in a process where "social facts . . . consist of manners of acting, thinking and feeling *external to the individual* . . . [and which] *exercise control over him*" (1982a, 52). Second, Durkheim never says, explicitly, that once under such "control," individuals proactively and interpretively *feedback* their now socially controlled "acting, thinking and feeling" into the group's *next* exercise of "control" over its individual participants (but see 1978, 130). In this way, the control of social facts over individual facts does not stop there but goes on to produce the influence that individual facts reciprocally exert over social facts—thereby producing the self-maintenance of both social facts and individual facts.

For example, Durkheim says "it is clear that the general characteristics of human nature play their part in the work of elaboration from which social life results." But he immediately minimizes the importance of that "part": "it is not these [general characteristics] which produce or give [social life] its special form: they only make [that form] possible. Collective representations, emotions and tendencies have not as their causes certain states of consciousness of individuals . . . [the real causes are] the conditions under which the body social as a whole exists" (1982a, 130–131). "The body social as a whole," then, *really* causes itself according to Durkheim. The individual human only mechanically *reacts* to the causal conditions that social facts impose on them—as billiard balls react to punches from an external cue-stick.

In making these claims, Durkheim ignores not only his own personal creative behavior in writing, say, *The Division of Labor*, but what he must also have known very well—namely, that many *non*human animals manifest sociocultural phenomena (see his reference to Alfred Victor Espinas's *Des Sociétés Animales* [1977, 308]), and that the genotypical behavior capabilities of the specifically *human* organism must play crucial roles in human sociocultural phenomena, just as genotypical *termite* behavior capabilities play crucial roles in termite social phenomena.

Durkheim, however, says nothing about the genotypically human *productive* physical capabilities that Marx emphasizes, or the genotypically human *interpretive* psychical capabilities that Weber emphasizes. Instead, Durkheim allocates to the human individual only a mechanical role in closing what he regards as a purely *sociocultural-to-sociocultural* circuit. We shall see in chapter 3 that Marx gives us a fuller portrait of proactive human *physical* behavior, and in chapter 4 that Weber gives us a fuller portrait of proactive human *psychical* behavior.

Durkheim's theory, however, taken as a whole, confronts four questions to which he devotes one book each: (1) What are the basic sociocultural mechanisms that hold a human society together during its two evolutionary stages and during the pivotal transition from the first to the second stage (*The Division of Labor in Society*, 1893)? (2) What can go wrong with these mechanisms (*Suicide*, 1897)? (3) Where did these mechanisms come from (*The Elementary Forms of Religious Life*, 1912)? (4) What is the likely future of these mechanisms (*Moral Education*, 1925)?

## *The Division of Labor in Society*

Durkheim's first major substantive work was his doctoral dissertation, subtitled *A Study of the Organization of Superior Societies*. (By "*superior*" societies" he meant, with the now-regrettable ethnocentrism of his time and place, and ours too, post–Industrial Revolution societies.) It is a largely speculative analysis of the evolution of human society from a simple to a complex stage. The simple stage is marked by what Durkheim calls a "segmentary" social structure ("division of labor") supported by a "mechanical" culture structure ("social solidarity"), and the complex stage is marked by what he calls an "organized" division of labor and an "organic" "social solidarity."

Durkheim credits Adam Smith with having been "the first to attempt to elaborate the theory of [the division of labor]" (1984, 1). But there are at least three differences between Smith's argument and Durkheim's:

First, Smith is interested only in the impact of the division of labor on the economic organizations. Durkheim, however, asserts that "the division of labor is *not peculiar to economic life*. . . . Functions, whether political, administrative or judicial [and we would add, religious, and informational], are becoming more specialized" (1984, 2).

Second, Smith tells us that "the effects of the division of labor" are "the greatest improvement in the *productive powers of [economic] labor*" (1937, 3), but Durkheim says "the most notable effect of the division of labor is not that it increases the productivity of . . . functions . . . but that it *links them very closely together*" (1984, 21).

Third, Smith argues that when the division of labor is at a *high*, complex level, the individual "intends only *his own* security . . . intends only *his own* gain, and he is . . . led by an *invisible hand* [we would say he is led by many, sometimes cross-cutting, sociocultural influences arising from his many institutional and organizational participations] to promote an end which was no part of his original intention. . . . By pursuing *his own* interest he frequently promotes [the interest] *of the society* more effectually than when he really intends to promote it" (1937, 423). Durkheim, however, correlates inversely individual psychical self-interest and sociocultural division of labor, citing Darwin (so we know that Durkheim read Darwin) to the effect that "two organisms *vie* with each other more keenly the more *alike* they are . . . [and] if each happens to increase in number in such proportions that all appetites can no longer be sufficiently assuaged, war breaks out." However, Durkheim continues, "The situation is totally different if the individuals coexisting together are of *different* species or varieties. As they do not feed in the same way or lead the same kind of life, they do not impede one another" (1984, 208–209), and so do not compete or conflict with one another.

Indeed, Durkheim tells us that such different individuals positively aid each other: "Individuals are linked to one another who would otherwise be independent. . . . They are solidly linked to one another and the links between them function not only in the brief moments when they engage in an exchange of services, but extend considerably beyond" (1984, 21).[3]

Thus it happens, Durkheim says (still following Darwin), that "In the same town *different* occupations can coexist without being forced into a position where they harm one another, for they are pursuing different objectives. The soldier seeks military glory, the priest moral authority, the statesman power, the industrialist wealth, the scientist professional fame" (1984, 209). (It seems only because Durkheim persistently overlooks the fact that the priest, the statesman, the industrialist, and the scientist are all living *individual human organisms* with the same psychical endowments that he overlooks that they *all* seek *all* of these benefits of participation in *all* the relevant organizations.)

The sociocultural evolutionary question, then, that Durkheim asks (implicitly) in *The Division of Labor* is: How is it possible that the simplest, low division of labor, type of human society, dominated by *generalist*-participants, could transform itself into the complex, high division of labor, *specialist*-dominated type of society, and sustain itself as such—just as Darwin had asked how it is possible that a single generalist, primeval species of life could transform itself into the millions of specialized species that now inhabit Earth.

Chapter 1 indicated that Darwin's answer to his question relies on the dividing migration of *whole organisms* to different geographical *habitats* followed by their descendants' further division (speciation) there. Durkheim's answer to *his* question, however, relies on the migration of *behaviors* from the *repertories* of participants as generalists to the repertories of participants as specialists in a society—followed by the development of a culture structural morality that regulates the exchanges among these now specialist participants in the same society so that none exploits any others.

## *Two Mechanisms of Human Societal Self-Maintenance: The Division of Labor and Social Solidarity*

Our basis, in that last paragraph, for subsuming Durkheim's terms, "division of labor" and "social solidarity," under broader terms that he himself does not use—namely, the terms social structure and culture structure (discussed in chapter 1) is as follows. Durkheim presents the "division of labor" as *social* structure when he refers to that division as *"physiological"* (rather than psychological) and says it is "the sharing out of *functions*" (1984, 83, 218)—while defining "functions" as "living *movements*" (1984, 11) and as "ways of *acting*" (1984, 302).[4] On the other hand, he presents "social solidarity" as "states of *consciousness*" that consist of collective *"sentiments"* (1984, 24; 1951, 381), thereby clearly implying its culture structurality.[5]

Simple human societies, according to Durkheim, have social structures with low divisions of labor (which he calls *"segmentary"* [see 1984, 132]—each segment having internal parts but being the same overall as other segments) and their own type of culture structural social solidarity (which he calls "mechanical"). Complex human societies have high divisions of labor (which he calls *"organ*ized") and their own type of culture structural social solidarity (which he calls "organic").[6]

Human society as a whole in both the evolutionary stages hypothesized by Durkheim, then, is *sociocultural*—never social structural alone and never culture structural alone—and the two structures, he claims, coevolve.[7] The question arises, however: which structure was originally cause and which was effect? (At first, we thought that at least some of the inconsistencies in Durkheim's answer to this question would have originated in translating the English from the French, but on comparing the two versions—we cite both below—we have found that all of the inconsistencies are present in Durkheim's original French.)

## *Which Is Cause and Which Is Effect?*

Durkheim asserts, even on the very same page, *both* causal directions between division of labor and social solidarity. Thus, on the one hand, he says that "solidarity *brings about* the division of labor," but on the other hand, and without so much as blinking an eye, he also says that "solidarity . . . is *due to* the division of labor" (1984, 85; cf. 1986a, 100–101).

No less unfortunately, however, Durkheim also uses the "division of labor" and "solidarity" as though they were synonyms referring to the same empirical datum when he asks: "whilst the division of labor is a law of [physical] nature, *is it also a [psychical] moral rule* for human conduct?" (1984, 3; cf. 1986a, 4); when he says we can compare the division of labor "with *other moral phenomena*" (1984, 6; cf. 1986a, 8); and when he claims that "it is the [physical] division of labor that is increasingly fulfilling the role that once fell to the [psychical] common consciousness" (1984, 123; cf. 1986a, 148). Having no explication from Durkheim, these seem to be logically inexplicable confusions on his part, and since they are present in the original French, we simply point them out and move on.

So let us now ask what, in Durkheim's view, *initiated* the simple "segmentary" division of labor—assuming that "mechanical" solidarity only comes into play to *maintain* that division after it was initiated. First, Durkheim says, "every aggregate of *individuals in continuous contact forms a society*" (1984, 218)—and to this we ourselves would add that that "continuous contact" must last long enough for the participant-intake, -organizing, and -outlet institutions that chapter 1 posited as constitutive of a "society: to be formed. Otherwise the "aggregate of individuals" in question would fall apart. But what accounts for the *initial* "contact"? Durkheim answers that "what draws men together are mechanical forces and instinctive forces such as the affinity of blood, attachment to the same soil, the cult of their ancestors, a [perceived] commonality of habits, etc." (1984, 219), and to that we can only say that every one of these "forces" appears to us distinctly *learned psychical consequences* of prior contact, not exogenous causes of subsequent contact.

At any rate, however, one possible consequence of first contact among wandering humans might be a simple division of labor (Durkheim calls it "segmentary") as, say, when one individual lifts one end of a log and another individual lifts the other end, followed by both individuals' shared thought that, because they can do more together than separately, they "belong" together (Durkheim calls these unifying thoughts "mechanical solidarity"). This early unison, or near-unison, interaction, Durkheim says, was broken down not by the rising population pressure on subsistence that Malthus had already claimed but by "the internal movements that develop within the mass of people, when this mass has been constituted" (1984, 219; Durkheim does not suggest what form these change-initiating "internal movements" might take).

Then, again, rather than calling on Malthus's population restraint as a mechanism to control these "internal movements," Durkheim argues that *"where the sentiment of solidarity [culture structure] is too weak* to resist the centrifugal influence of [social structural] competition . . . [and in] countries where existence is too difficult because of the extreme [physical] density of the population, *the inhabitants, instead of specializing, withdraw permanently or provisionally from [their] society by emigrating to other areas"* (1984, 217)—as Darwin (whom Durkheim does cite) proposed. Durkheim's next two sentences offer a strikingly vague explanation for the division of labor. "It is enough," he says, "to represent to ourselves what the division of labor is to make us understand that things cannot be otherwise [but he claims they *were* otherwise!]. It consists in the sharing out of functions that up until then were common to all" (1984, 217–218).

Durkheim, then, goes on to argue that if the sentiment of solidarity is neither too strong nor too weak but *just right* (as he argues it would be given communication between parties who already know each other as participants in segmentary social structure and mechanical culture structure; see 1984, 218), then not Darwin's geographical migration (division of place) but Smith's division of labor will initiate its own organic culture structural solidarity.

In short, where the "mechanical" type of solidarity (culture structure) supported the "segmentary" type of division of labor (social structure) by prescribing the *same* behavior to and from everyone—that is, "do unto *all* others as you would have them *all* do unto you"—the "organic" type of solidarity supports the "organized" type of division of labor by prescribing *different* physical and psychical behaviors to and from participants who perform *different* functions. That is to say, "organic" solidarity tells participants "do unto *particular others as their different occupational specialties would have you do unto them.*" It seems that this is why Durkheim tells us "there are as many forms of morals as there are different callings" (1992, 3, 4, 5; see also 110).

But, one asks, what holds a society together during its disintegration-threatening transition from "segmentary" division of labor to "organized" division of labor? Durkheim tells us this integrator is a residual amount of "mechanical" solidarity, for, he says, "nowhere is organic solidarity to be met with in isolation [presumably, from mechanical solidarity]" (1984, 138; cf. Giddens 1979, 34–35)—which is to say, there is always some minimal mechanical solidarity holding together every human society. Although "in the more advanced societies, the similarities that are required are *fewer* in number" (1984, 329), still *some* moral similarities are required even in those societies, for "*society can survive only if there exists among its members a sufficient degree of homogeneity*" (1956, 70; see also 1973a, 87–88)—which seems to be the same sort of general culture structural cohesiveness (not adhesiveness) that Giddings calls "consciousness of kind" (1896, 17–18), that Cooley calls "we-feeling" (1956, 189–190), and that Ibn Khaldûn calls "group feeling" (see chapter 5).

This persistent culture structural sense of homogeneity is so essential to a human society's continuation in Durkheim's eyes that he tells us that "the division of labor cannot be carried out save between the members of a society already constituted. Indeed when competition opposes isolated individuals *not known to one another*, it can only separate them still more" (1984, 217). And note that Durkheim's very unusual mention of "individuals" here implies they have roles in simple societies as well as complex societies. We indicate this role in our summary of

*The Division of Labor in Society* as shown in figure 2.1 by including there a causal factor that we call "*individual* behavior." This factor is sometimes connected only by implication (dashed arrows) to the level called "*collective* behavior" in Durkheim's theory but it is, we claim, always a necessary constituent of sociocultural phenomena.

It is, then, a persistent cultural *consensus* about the generalized *we*-ness among individual members of a society (in contrast with the alienating *them*-ness that those members implicitly attribute to members of *other* societies) that acts as a collective cocoon inside which that segmentary social division of labor, Durkheim says, "vanishes" while "organized" division of labor begins to grow its own "organic" social solidarity (1984, 132, 136, 138, 200).

Eventually, then, within the evolving society, three factors—residual mechanical solidarity, the new organized division of labor, and the emergent organic solidarity which the latter sponsors—co-evolve to replace the older stage of sociocultural evolution with a new, stably self-maintaining, high division of labor stage (see 1984, 122, 132–138, 218).

## Quantitative Abnormalities in Sociocultural Self-Maintenance

In book 3 of *The Division of Labor*, Durkheim raises what is, from our point of view, a key diagnostic, *forecasting*, question—namely, what could go *wrong* with the sociocultural evolution he has indicated? What, in other words, could lead to a society's *termination* instead of its partial self-*maintenance*?

Thus, labeling as "pathological" any "*organized*" division of labor that fails to engender its own appropriately "organic" social solidarity (see 1984, 291)—because, he says, "there is no form of [human] social activity which can do without the appro-

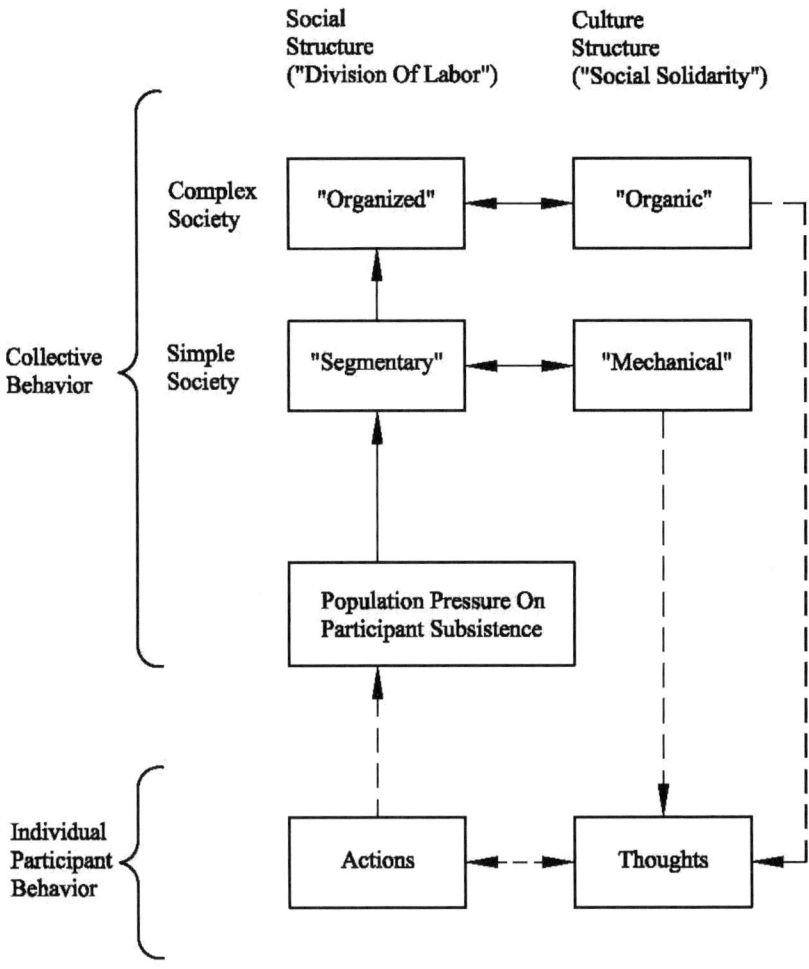

Figure 2.1. Durkheim's *The Division of Labor in Society*

priate moral discipline" (1992, 14)—Durkheim tells us that "if *normally* the division of labor produces [the appropriate] social solidarity, it can happen . . . that [the division of labor] has entirely different or even opposite [that is, *abnormal*] results" (1984, 291).

Durkheim therefore proposes three *abnormal* forms of the "organized" division of labor, which he names "anomic," "forced," and (with altogether regrettable vagueness) "another." The first abnormal form, called "*anomic*"—that is, literally *normless*, without *rules, amoral*—seems to be the type-case of the "organized" division of labor's nonproduction of its appropriate culture structural social solidarity. But what would explain that nonproduction? In answer, Durkheim tells us that such a "state of anomie is impossible wherever organs solidly linked to one another are in sufficient *contact*, and in sufficiently lengthy *contact*" (1984, 304). Therefore (setting aside that Durkheim does not define "solidly" or "sufficiently"), it would seem that Durkheim might better have named this abnormality "*insufficient [physical] contact*" to underscore that this pathology originates in the social structural division of labor and not in its cultural structural solidarity—as one might well have been misled to think by Durkheim's misnaming it anomic—which is to say "normless."

Calling the second abnormality in the division of labor the "*forced*" form, Durkheim says that "the [physical] distribution of social functions [among individuals] . . . does not correspond, or rather no longer corresponds, to the distribution of natural abilities [among them]" (1984, 311 see also 1986c, 49–50)—which is to say, there exists a *discriminatory* social structure leading to a *systematic mismatch of participants' talents to their tasks in the division of labor*.

In describing the third (loosely, "another") form of abnormality, Durkheim locates it, too, in the division of labor when he tells us that here "activities are *badly coordinated* and operations are carried out *without concertation*" (1984, 323), so it would have been more informative to have called this form "inadequate coordination."

Nevertheless, it seems fair to say that all three abnormal forms discussed in *The Division of Labor* are indeed located in the social structural *division of labor*, and all three forms are *deficiencies* there—that is, too little contact among tasks; too little person-to-task efficiency; and too little coordination among tasks and persons. Such abnormalities, however, logically imply their symmetry partners—namely, that abnormalities may originate *in culture structural solidarity* as well as in the social structural division of labor; and they may be manifested in *excesses* as well as deficiencies in the indicated qualities of both mechanisms. Durkheim investigates these implications in his next book, *Suicide*, although unfortunately he does not tell us that is what he is doing, nor does he tell us how the indicated shortcomings might be remedied.

Before leaving *The Division of Labor in Society*, however, let us suggest a title for that book that summarizes our view of it as part 1 of a larger series—namely, *The Division of Labor in Society, Part 1: Social Structural and Culture Structural Mechanisms of Human Societal Self-Maintenance, and Some Possible Abnormalities Therein.*[8]

## *Suicide*

The only thing Durkheim reveals about any theory that may underlie his second book, *Suicide,* is that "from every page [of *Suicide*] . . . the impression [will emerge] that *the individual is dominated by a moral reality greater than himself: namely, collective reality*" (1951, 36–37, 38), which echoes his definition of a "social fact": "a social fact [we would say a sociocultural phenomenon] is identifiable *through the power of external coercion* [domination] *which it exerts or is capable of exerting upon individuals*" (1982a, 56). "Social facts," then, include the power to induce human individuals to take their own lives, thereby injuring both the human sociocultural structure and the human species.

However, still overlooking the proactive human participant in human sociocultural phenomena, Durkheim again *omits the individual feedback* component of his definition of such phenomena, the component that would complete his sociocultural *self-maintenance* hypothesis. Clearly, this hypothesis requires attention not only to "*the power of external coercion* which [the social fact] exerts or is capable of exerting upon individuals" but also to *the power of feedback* which the suicidal individual exerts on the social fact called "suicide"—and eventually on human species survival.

## Social Structure "Integration" and Culture Structure "Regulation"

The theoretical relationship of *Suicide* to *The Division of Labor* is more intimate than that, however, for *Suicide* also generalizes and renames the two self-maintenance mechanisms Durkheim introduced in *The Division of Labor* (namely, "division of labor" and "social solidarity"), as "integration" and "regulation," and examines their bearing on the opposite of sociocultural self-maintenance—that is, on sociocultural self-*termination*.

Thus, Durkheim tells us that "the state of *integration* of a social aggregate can only reflect the intensity of the collective life circulating in it. It is more unified and powerful the more active and constant is the intercourse among its members" (1951, 202, see also 217)—thereby implying the social structural nature of "integration." He also states that "a *regulative force can only be moral*" (1951, 249; see also 276)—thereby even more clearly indicating that "regulation" is culture structural. His research hypothesis is that certain states of "integration" and "regulation" increase the rate at which individual societal participants choose to *exit* from their own society and from the possibility of entering any other society. *Suicide,* then, represents the converse of *The Division of Labor*'s asking why individuals *enter and remain in* a society and it finds, basically, the same answer, reversed, as does *The Division of Labor.*

At the same time, however, *The Division of Labor* and *Suicide* differ from each other in at least three essential ways. The first difference is that *The Division of Labor* focuses on explaining actions that only *collectivities* can carry out, while *Suicide* focuses on actions that only *individuals* can carry out. That is to say, it takes a *collectivity* to manifest the division of labor and social solidarity, but only *individual persons* can manifest suicide—otherwise it is murder.

Second, where *The Division of Labor* bears on the participant-*organizing* institution of society and its organizations, *Suicide* bears on phenomena that render individuals objects for the participant-*outlet* institution and its cadaver-managing organizations. Suicide can have increasingly profound consequences for the persistence of human society and the human species as the numbers of suicides mount up to larger and larger proportions of a population. Durkheim himself says that "what the rising flood of voluntary deaths denotes is . . . a *state of crisis and perturbation* [of the society] not to be prolonged with impunity" (1951, 369; see also 1984, lv). But why should such an act be "of interest to the *sociologist*. . . . [Its study would seem to belong] to *psychology alone*. Is not the suicide's resolve usually explained by his [personal] temperament, [personal] character, [personal] antecedents and private history?" (1951, 46).[9] But true to his claim that "*Social facts* consist of manners of acting, thinking and feeling . . . [that] *exercise control over* [*the individual*]," and the still unspoken implication that the controlled individual is then influenced to join, and thereby strengthen, the *next* exercise of such control over individuals, Durkheim diagnoses every human society as being "*predisposed to contribute a definite quota of voluntary deaths*" (1951, 51) to the termination of that society and to the termination of all human societies.

## *Moderation as Quantitative Mechanism of Societal Self-Maintenance*

The third difference that sets *Suicide* apart from *The Division of Labor* is more method than content. Where *The Division of Labor* claims only *linear* relationships (for example, Durkheim says that "the division of labor only produces solidarity . . . to the degree that it is spontaneous" [1984, 312, italics removed; see also 304, 323]), *Suicide* makes the nonlinear, moderationist, claim that *too strong* as well as *too weak* relationships dispose human individual sociocultural participants to take their own lives. Thus, Durkheim tells us both that *excessive* social structural "integration" and *excessive* culture structural "regulation" (conditions that he calls "altruistic" and "fatalistic," respectively—see 1951, 276), as well as *deficient* levels of those variables (called "egoistic" and "anomic") are powerful influences toward individual self-destruction. In sum, "when [a] man has become *detached* from society," Durkheim says, "he encounters less resistance to suicide in himself, and he does so likewise when social integration is *too strong*" (1951, 217; see also 258).

Therefore Durkheim tells us "there is a type of suicide the *opposite* of anomic suicide, just as egoistic and altruistic suicides are *opposites*" (1951, 276).[10] Now we know that "egoistic and altruistic suicides are opposites" insofar as the first results from *deficient integration* and the second results from *excessive integration*, so the type that Durkheim says is "the opposite of anomic suicide" (which results from *deficient regulation*) must result from *excessive regulation*. Durkheim refers to this latter type ("fatalistic" suicide) only once in all of *Suicide* (1951, 276), and then only in a brief footnote—thereby suggesting that this type of suicide (and even Durkheim's moderationism in general) may have been an after-typesetting-realization rather than part of Durkheim's originating conceptualization of this work.

## Society and the Individual Participant

Next, turning to examine the suicidal *individual*, Durkheim says that "when [the individual's] *resolution* entails certain sacrifice of life, scientifically this is suicide" (1951, 44). So psychical resolve (that is, strong, end-focused desire) to die by one's own hand must be followed by physical commission of an act that one psychically knows will satisfy that resolve: "the term suicide is applied to all cases of death resulting directly or indirectly from a positive or negative *[physical] act* of the victim himself, which he [psychically, and deterministically] knows *will* produce this result" (1951, 44). So now we have two psychical behaviors that Durkheim proposes as susceptible to sociocultural influence, and that produce suicide: one is the individual's "*desire*" to exit from life; the second is the individual's deterministic *forecast* that certain of her/his own acts *"will* produce this result." Apart from making the latter, as all human forecasts, probabilistic, we would add a third behavior that Durkheim omits—namely, scientifically educated *know-how* regarding the technique of effective manifestation of the "positive or negative act of the victim himself" so that the desired result is, in fact, likely to be produced.

To all this, Durkheim implicitly adds a fourth factor—namely, the physical *opportunity* to perform suicide—when he cites "the totality of customs and usages of all kinds [that put] one *instrument* of death rather than another at [an individual's] disposal," pointing out that such differential physical opportunity "is why suicides by throwing one's self from a high place are oftener committed in great cities than in the country: the buildings are higher" (1951, 292).[11]

So Durkheim suggests (but unfortunately for us readers, not all in one place) that in order to commit suicide an individual must have the *physical opportunity* to employ at least one effective geographical and/or technological instrument to that end, the *psychical desire* to use that instrument, the *psychical belief* that she or he can fulfill that desire through that instrument, and the *psychical know-how* regarding the exact manner the instrument can be operated to make the desired result likely. All these factors, Durkheim says, are liable to "the power of external coercion" that define "social facts."

Now among Durkheim's many formulations of the sociocultural self-maintenance proposition is the bald assertion that *"once the individual is ruled out, only society remains.* It is therefore in the nature of *society* itself that we must seek the explanation of social life" (1982a, 128). We point out here only one implication of this statement which leaves out the entire rest of the universe—namely, that if "the individual" were *not* "ruled out," we would have to include some *explanatory power of that "individual" over "social life."* Therefore, because he does not *completely* rule out the proactive individual, Durkheim implicitly allows that one individual suicide's physically manifested cognitive *knowledge and know-how* of suicidal acts may become a "social fact" that pressures ("coerces") potential suicidal individuals to see themselves as "gathered together" in the same logical category of sharing that knowledge and know-how—with each other and with the first individual. "A sort of electricity [can then be] generated from their closeness [that] quickly launches [the still-living, knowing, individuals] to an extraordinary height of exaltation" (1995, 217). At that point, one may hypothesize the possible emergence of a sociocultural *movement* feeding back, abnormally, toward societal self-*termination* rather than toward societal self-maintenance.

In summary of *Suicide*, then, we propose figure 2.2, together with a tentative retitling that sees that work as *The Division of Labor, Part 2: The Suicide Rate, Empirical Indicator of Quantitative Abnormalities in the Social Structural and Culture Structural Mechanisms of Human Societal Self-Maintenance.*[12]

## *The Elementary Forms of Religious Life*

Whereas, as we shall see in chapter 3, Marx applauds the development of a cultural structure within each socioeconomic class (i.e., "class consciousness") that calls for conflict, not cooperation, with the other class, Durkheim sees such conflict as a default eventuality that is due to the *absence* of norms: "It is to [the] state of *anomie* that . . . must be attributed the continually recurring *conflicts* and disorder of every kind of which the economic world affords so sorry a spectacle. For, since nothing re-

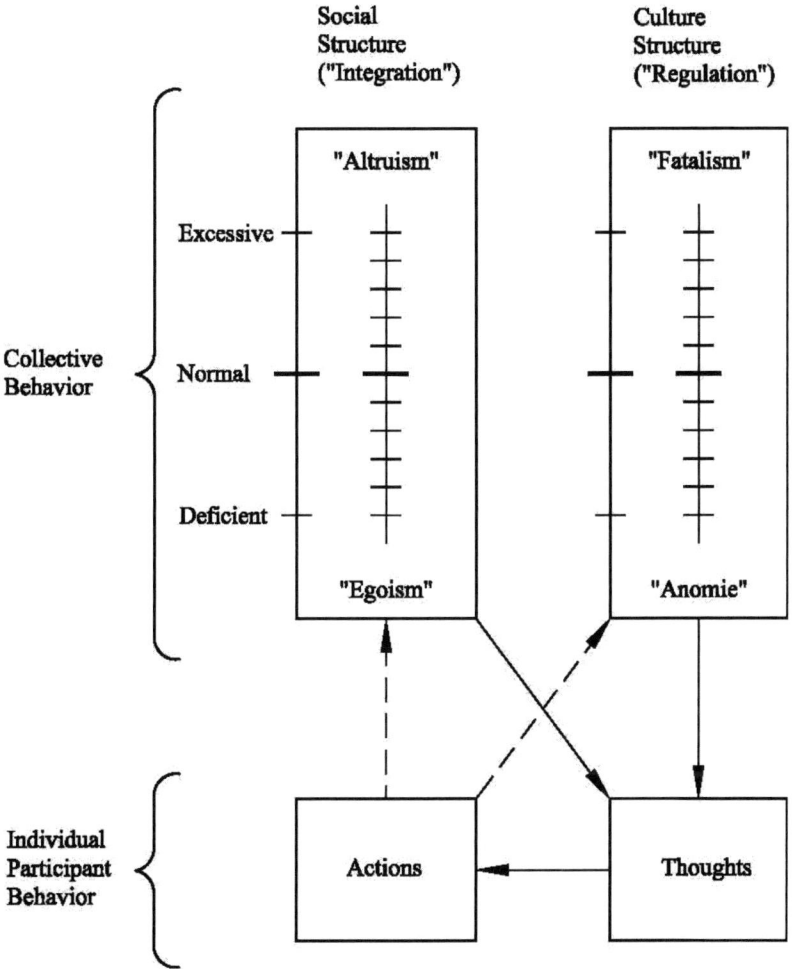

Figure 2.2. Durkheim's *Suicide*

strains the forces present from reacting together . . . they tend to grow beyond all bounds, each clashing with the other, each warding off and weakening the other" (1984, xxxii). "If [moral] authority . . . is *lacking*," he says, "it is the law of the *strongest* that rules, and a state of warfare, either latent or acute, is necessarily endemic" (1984, xxxii–xxxiii). Marx is more succinct in making the same point: "between equal rights *force* decides" (1967, 1:235), for where there are no norms, there can be no rights.

## Mediation Added to Moderation

In addition to a moral culture structure, Durkheim says, a society needs social structures: "A nation *cannot be maintained unless, between the state and individuals, a whole range of secondary groups [is] interposed* [Durkheim neither defines nor instantiates a 'primary' group]. These must be close enough to the individual to attract him strongly to their activities and, in so doing, to absorb him into the mainstream of social life" (1984, liv). Durkheim refers to economic organizations as "corporations" and says they should have "assemblies . . . [that] should clearly include representatives of employees and employers . . . [and these two should] constitute *distinct and independent groups* at the lowest level of corporative organization because too often their interests vie with one another and are opposing" (1984, lix)—a meaty bone to Marx.

By contrast, in religious organizations, "*beliefs and practices* [culture structures and social structures] . . . *unite into one single moral community called a Church, all those who adhere to them*" (1995, 44, italics augmented), and "rites are ways of *acting* [social structures] that are born only in the midst of assembled groups and whose purpose is to evoke, maintain, or recreate certain *mental states* [culture structures] of those groups" (1995, 9).[13] Spatial proximity, then, sustains rites, which sustains that proximity, which also sustains beliefs, which feed back to sustain rites: "The essence of the [elementary religious] cult is the cycle of [social structural] *feasts* that are regularly repeated at definite times. . . . Society cannot revitalize the [culture structural] *awareness* that it has of itself unless it [social structurally] *assembles*, but it cannot remain continuously in session. The demands of life do not permit [it] to stay in congregation indefinitely, so it disperses, only to reassemble anew when it again feels the need" (1995, 353; see also 59–60).

## From Social Structural Contact to Extraordinary Culture Structural Communication

One might think that the regularity of spatial assembly would eventually render it boringly ho-hum to their participants, but Durkheim tells us that the spatial closeness of participants in the congregations *always stimulates extraordinary forms of communication* (which "forms" he and Weber both call "contagion," and Simmel calls "mass excitement" [see 1955, 217–220, 328–329; 1978, 23, 1377; 1950, 36]; cf. Miller et al. 1960, 25–27; Berger and Luckmann 1967, 56). As partly quoted above, Durkheim says "once the individuals are gathered together, a sort of electricity is generated from their closeness and quickly launches them to an extraordinary height of exaltation . . . it is as if [the individual were] in reality transported into a special world entirely different from the one in which he ordinarily lives, a special world inhabited by exceptionally intense forces that invade and transform him" (1995, 217, 220; see also Parsons 1949, 435, 436, 439; Collins 1994, 232–234).

In short, "the people of a totem," Durkheim says, "cannot remain themselves unless the people *periodically renew* the totemic principle that is in them" (1995, 342). Thus: "a cult . . . is a system of rites, feasts, and various ceremonies all having the characteristic that *they recur, periodically.* They meet the need that the faithful feel periodically to tighten and strengthen the bond between them and the sacred beings on which they depend" (1995, 59–60; see also 353, 420).

In sum, "the effect of the cult is [to bring about spatial proximity among its participants] periodically [and thus] to recreate a moral being on which we depend, as it depends upon us," and "this being exists: It is society" (1995, 352). Religious cults, then, are the organizational producers of human societies. Without such periodic ceremonial congregation, the sense of extraordinariness that repeatedly refuels individuals' sense of their shared personal sacredness would eventually be forgotten. With it, however, the world becomes collectively partitioned between cult congregation times and cult dispersion times—that is, "into two domains, one containing all that is *sacred* and the other all that is *profane*"—one domain that is *in* Sabbaths and another that is *between* Sabbaths. This cyclical togetherapartness, congregation-individuation, becomes "the distinctive trait of religious thought" (1995, 34).

Although Durkheim himself does not tell us, the crucial faculty of "religious thought" seems to be that it confers sacred *honor and self-confidence on every individual participant in the cult assembly*—while nonparticipating individuals (typically women, children, old people, and, most importantly, all individuals belonging to other societies and therefore to other religious organizations—see 1995, 384) are permitted to have only low honor, no honor, or dishonor.[14]

Durkheim is quite explicit (and extreme) regarding the *fact* of this separation of domains (he does not consider the possibility of a sociocultural world—say a monastery or nunnery—that is regarded as *entirely* sacred, or *entirely* profane): "the sacred and the profane are *always* and *everywhere* conceived by the human intellect as separate genera, as two worlds with *nothing* in common. . . . Indeed, this heterogeneity is such that it degenerates into real antagonism. The two worlds are conceived of not only as separate, but also as hostile and jealous rivals" (1995, 36). Thus, "Sacred things," Durkheim says, "are things *protected and isolated* by prohibitions; profane things are those things to which the prohibitions are applied " (1995, 37).

Durkheim adds, crucially to that definition, however, when he tells us that sacred things "tend to be regarded as *superior* in dignity and power to profane things"—even though "*subordination* of one thing to another is not enough to make one sacred and the other not" (1995, 35). So it is not necessarily superiority but what we would call *extraordinariness*—that is, the "*extraordinary* height of exaltation," and its "contagion"—that makes the participant in religious congregations feel transported into "a *special* world inhabited by *exceptionally* intense forces that invade and transform him." Feeling that one has the honor and self-confidence of such extraordinary experience marks the sacred (see Goleman 1991)—and marks, therefore, full-fledged members of one's own society but not members of other, or no, society.[15]

But one can hardly help noticing Durkheim's reluctance to discuss how extraordinariness (and its derivative "sacredness") is *defined* in a given society, although he takes pains to state how it is *not* defined: "Sacred things," he says, "are *not* simply those personal beings that are called gods or spirits. A rock, a tree, a spring, a pebble, a piece of wood, a house, in a word *anything*, can be sacred" (1995, 34–35). (We shall meet this "anything" idea again in Weber's concept of charisma.) Moreover, Durkheim tells us that the "dignity and power" of the sacred does not need to be *super*natural—if we understand by that word a "world of mystery, the unknowable, or the incomprehensible" (1995, 22; cf. Pickering 2000, 78; Jones 1998, 39).

In any case, however, the result of the sacred–profane partitioning is a culture structural segregation that reinforces the protection of experiences, people, and things that are thought to be extraordinary and sacred from loss of their "dignity and power" to ordinary and profane experiences, people, and things. And once this protective quarantine becomes culture structurally rule-bound and symbolically represented in a totem, its presence and perception generates powerful psychical bonds among cult participants—bonds that obligate the giving of assistance, mourning, and vengeance in defending the memory of their common ancestors, their common possessions, their common customs, their common society.

Then it is, Durkheim concludes, that social structural "acts of worship . . . [serve] the manifest purpose of strengthening the [culture structural] ties *between the faithful and their god*—the god being only a figurative representation of the *society*—[which in turn strengthens both the physical and the psychical] . . . ties *between the individual and the society* of which he is a member" (1995, 227; contrast Bellah 1973, ix–x), which by strengthening the individual's contribution to the society, ensures the society's—and the species'—self-maintenance. Thus do the divine right of kings and the kingly right of gods join hands in defense of their society in two worlds.

## The Societal Self-Maintenance Role of Religious Organizations

Durkheim tells us that he "would like to find a means of discerning the *ever-present causes* on which the most basic forms of religious thought and practice depend. . . . [Such] causes are more easily observable if the societies in which they are observed are less complex. That," he says, "is *why I seek to get closer to the origins*" (1995, 7). Durkheim, then, wants "to get closer to the *origins*" in order to find causes that he believes are operating in the *present,* and will operate in the *future*—a strong manifestation of his causal determinism (discussed in chapter 6), which overlooks entirely the possibility of an evolutionary succession of different *substitute* causes that serve the same persistent effect.

So let us ask, as we did when considering his views of society as a whole, which comes first in Durkheim's view of the religious organizations: *material* ties or *moral* ties among the participants—social structure or culture structure? We ask this question again because we suspect that in *The Elementary Forms of the Religious Life* Durkheim may not *only* be undertaking the specific task he says he is undertaking—namely, "to study the simplest and most primitive *religion* that is known at present, [in order to] discover *its* principles and attempt an explanation of *it*" (1995, 1; see Hunt 1988, 26). He may also—even mainly—be trying to answer how a fortuitous and ordinarily passing contact among wandering human kin groups could have become "continuous" enough to get not only religion and its periodic assemblies started but the ancestors of *all* human participant-organizing, as well as participant-intake, and participant-outlet, societal institutions started.

He may, in short, be trying to discern "the *ever*-present [original] causes" of human society as a whole.

Consider again, then, Durkheim's argument that "collective life awakens religious thought when it rises to a certain intensity . . . because it brings about a state of effervescence that alters the conditions of psychic activity" (1995, 424): "because his companions [psychically] feel transformed in the same way at the same moment, and express this feeling [physically] by their shouts, movements, and bearing, it is as if he were in reality transported into a special world entirely different from the one in which he ordinarily lives" (1995, 217, 220).[16] Accordingly, Durkheim tells us that "religion is first and foremost a system of *ideas* [culture structure] by means of which individuals *imagine* the society of which they are members and the obscure yet intimate relations they have with it" but he also says that social structural "*acts* of worship . . . [which are visible to all congregants, by] strengthening the ties between the faithful and their god . . . at the same time strengthen the ties between the individual and the society of which [the individual] is a member" (1995, 271).

Not only do perceivable "acts of worship" strengthen culture structural ties *within* generations; they also strengthen ties *between* generations. Indeed, Durkheim tells us that "belief in the immortality of the soul is the *only* way man is able to comprehend . . . the perpetuity of the *group's* life. The individuals die, but the clan survives, so the forces that constitute his life must have the *same* perpetuity" (1995, 271; see also Fields 1996, 196–197). In this last remark about the individual's life being seen as having the same perpetuity as the clan's, we see the same determinism as when Durkheim tells us "to the same effect there always corresponds the same cause" (1982a, 150), discussed further in chapter 6. (But hasn't Durkheim just said the reverse—namely, that belief in the immortality of the individual soul is the only way we comprehend the perpetuity of the group?)

## The Continuous Demands of Secular Life and the Periodic Demands of Sacred Religious Congregation

A stressful threat, however, is imposed on the ties "between the faithful and their god" by factors such as the individual's secular psychophysical need for variety, subsistence, rest, sleep, but these intervening "down" times are spanned by collectively shared memories of the congregation's previous sacred "high" times and anticipations of the next high time.

As this together-apart-together-apart cycle accumulates and becomes traditional, Durkheim says, the culture structural regulation of participants' behaviors spreads from the imagined sacred world to the sensory profane world: "Sacredness is highly contagious and it spreads from the totemic being to everything that directly or remotely has to do with it" (1995, 224) (Durkheim offers no explanation for such contagion, but see chapter 4)—which would seem to be literally *everything* that humans perceive. Thus, Durkheim concludes, "the most disparate techniques and practices—those that ensure the continuity of moral life (law, morals, fine arts) and those that are useful to material life (natural sciences, industrial techniques)—sprang from religion, directly or indirectly" (1995, 225).[17] More than that, "there are certain fundamental notions that dominate our entire intellectual life. It is these ideas that philosophers, beginning with Aristotle, have called the categories of the understanding: notions of time, space, number, cause, substance, personality." All these ideas, Durkheim says, are "a *product of religious thought*" (1995, 8–9).

## Role of Religious Culture Structure in the Evolution toward Advanced Society

Having originated in the sacred religious organizations, these secular ideas are communicated to all the other participant-organizing organizations, where, in time, they eventually overcome the domination of society by religious organizations. Thus, gradually, "religion extends over an *ever-diminishing* area of social life" (1984, 119; see also 1995, 431).

In the consequently enlarging *non*religious, *profane*, areas of social life, Durkheim argues, the effect is humanizing: "there is no longer the same distance between the offender and the offended; they are more nearly on an equal footing. . . . The attack of a man against a man could not incite the same indignation of the attack of a man against a god" (1978, 174–175). In this way, *political egalitarianism* among societal participants finds a culture structural foothold—and this, Durkheim says, was "the great change which occurred in the course of moral evolution . . . [wherein] social discipline . . . loses more and more of its authoritarian vigor . . . [and] takes on more of a human character" (1978, 178; see also 1994, 194–195).

Supporting these two religion-sponsored but paradoxically religion-*diminishing* developments—namely, the emergence of empirically scientific information and of political egalitarianism—Durkheim argues, is the fitfully emerging *global consolidation* of individual societies. Thus, he says "a new kind of social life gradually developed: *international* life, whose effect . . . was to universalize religious beliefs. As that international life broadens, [an individual society] no longer appears as the whole . . . and becomes part of a whole that is more vast, with frontiers that are indefinite and capable of rolling back indefinitely" (1995, 446).

\*

In summary of *The Elementary Forms of the Religious Life*, let us propose its retitling as *The Division of Labor, Part 3: 'The Religious Organizations as Initiating and Maintaining Simple Societies and as Providing the Basis for the Culture Structure of Complex Societies*, together with figure 2.3. In this figure we again include dashed arrows to make explicit the individual participant's proactive role, which as claimed above, Durkheim always leaves unstated.

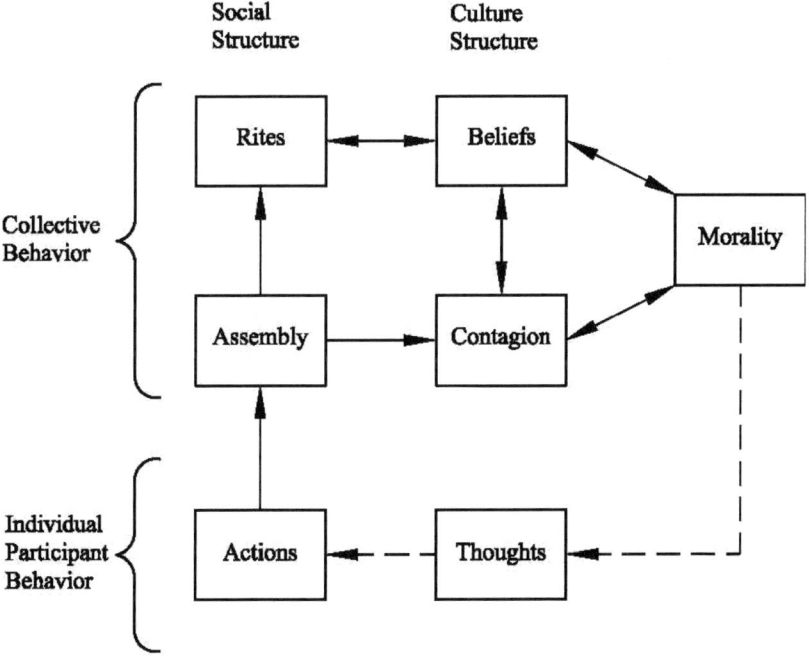

Figure 2.3. Durkheim's *The Elementary Forms of the Religious Life*

## Moral Education

The final substantive work of Durkheim's that we consider here also derives logically from his first such work, but in a different way from *Suicide*. Where *Suicide* diagnoses possible *abnormalities* in social structure and in culture structure that could undermine an entire society and therefore the species of its participants, *Moral Education* offers an analysis of how the culture structure of a society with a high division of labor should *normally* progress.

### From a Sacred Religious Morality to a Secular Scientific Morality

In modern societies, Durkheim says, "*education* must assure, among [all] the citizens, a sufficient community of ideas and of sentiments, without which any society is impossible" (1956 [1911], 80—referring to what we have called the cultural persistence of mechanical solidarity). The basis of these ideas and sentiments, he says, begins with their having a character set by *religious* organizations but evolves into a character set by the secular informational organizations—a change that marks the successful transition from simple to complex social structure and culture structure. Durkheim's concern here is only with teaching *moral* (that is, interpersonal conative, behavior preparatory) precepts—and he assumes that if such precepts are properly taught, they will also be properly learned and carried out. He expresses no slightest concern for teaching any cognitive or cathectic, or any other conative, precepts (see 1973a, 261–281).

Durkheim defines "morality" as "the sum of definite and special *rules* [culture structure] that *imperatively determine* [social structural] *conduct*" (1973a, 33), and he tells us that "the most essential element of [an individual's] character is this capacity for [imperative] *restraint* . . . which allows us to *contain* our passions, our desires, our habits, and subject them to law" (1973a, 46). That is, Durkheim assumes we all *possess* such passions either as part of our genotype or as part of our basic participant-intake socialization, but we must learn to restrain and reorient those passions in order to fulfill our participant-organizing roles. We learn to do this, Durkheim says, in accord with morality "because we *ought* to, regardless of the consequences our conduct may have for us. One must obey a moral precept out of *respect* for *it* and for this reason alone" (1973a, 30—Weber calls this respect "charisma" in chapter 4).

Now although Durkheim asserts that "there *is* no morality that is not infused with religiosity" (1960, 335; see also 1995, 214), he also says that a "morality *could* be constructed quite independent of any theological conception" and comments that if "ever a revolution has been a long time in the making, [the construction of such a religion-free morality] is it" (1973a, 7). Here, then, Durkheim tells us that "we must discover the rational *substitutes* for those religious notions that for a long time have served as the vehicle for the most essential moral ideas" (1973a, 9, see also 11)[18]—although he does not say why we "must" do so, nor does he acknowledge that discovering a "substitute" for anything, in principle, operates against his preferred causal determinism (discussed in chapter 6).

To achieve the indicated "substitution," Durkheim focuses only on the particular participant-intaking organization (primary school) that trains children to take up various adult roles in all the institutions and organizations of their societies because "society finds itself, with each new generation faced with a *tabula rasa*, very nearly, on which it must build anew. To the egoistic and asocial being that has just been born it must, as rapidly as possible, add another, capable of leading a moral and social life" (1956, 72; see also 125). Note the tacit connection to *Suicide* here: school teachers daily face populations of insufficiently integrated (egoistic) and insufficiently regulated (anomic) human individuals and must keep them from committing suicide, not to mention homicide. "Education is the influence exercised by adult cohorts on those that are not yet fully ready for social life. Its object is to arouse and to develop in the child a certain number of physical, intellectual and moral states [no mention of physical abilities] which are demanded of him by both the political society as a whole and the special milieu for which he is specifically destined" (1956, 71; see also 70).

Regarding two of the participant-intake organizations—family and school—that promulgate these states in the child, Durkheim tells us that "I judge that the task of the *school* is the moral development of the child . . . [and it] should be of the greatest importance . . . in terms of the demands of *society*" (1973a, 18–19; see also 144).

## *A Scientific Morality?*

Durkheim says that his aim in *Moral Education* "is not to formulate moral education for man *in general*; but for men of *our time in this country*" (1973a, 3), implying that moral education is likely to have evolved, and to be still evolving, and so to be different in other times and other places. The content of the time-and-place-specific education his book plans, he says, should have three parts. The first part combines "*regularity* [i.e., habitual obedience to rules] and . . . *authority*" (one person's expectation that another person will obey him/her and vice-versa) and "may be described as the spirit of *discipline*" (1973a,

35). The reason this spirit is called "moral" and not "disciplinary," Durkheim says, is that "*norms* must be established [in the population] which determine what proper relationships are, and to which people conform" (1973a, 37; see also 1956, 88) out of *respect* and not merely out of fear of punishment (but that, too?).

The second part of the morality the school should inculcate, Durkheim says, is "the individual's [psychical] *attachment to a group* of which he is a member" (1973a, 64). Note that Durkheim does not acknowledge the possibility of equally loyal attachments to *multiple,* sometimes even competing, groups. "There is no truly moral force," he says, "save that involved in attachment to *a* group" (1973a, 82). To this, Durkheim adds his rhetorical (and flawed) proposition that "morality is made *for* society. Is it not, then, a priori evident that it is made *by* society? . . . If a society is the end of morality, it is also its producer" (1973a, 85–86).

"*Society*," Durkheim claims, "is the end [that is, we hasten to add, not the termination but the goal] of morality," and "there never has existed any people among whom an *egoistic* act—that is to say, behavior directed solely to the interest of the person performing it—has been considered moral" (1973a, 57–58). But a few pages later Durkheim tells us that "one of the fundamental axioms of our morality—perhaps even the fundamental axiom—is that *the human being* is the sacred thing par excellence" (1973a, 107), which strikes a discordant note with "*society* is the end of morality."

In any event, however, Durkheim does not intend the paramount honorific status he has just given to the individual to entail political *freedom* to that individual: "to be free," Durkheim says, "is not to do what one pleases, it is to know how to act with *reason* and to do one's *duty*" (1956, 87, 89–90). In short, to be free one must be bound.

But what if duty and reason conflict? To avoid the possibility of such a conflict, Durkheim says that there is "a human science of morality [that shows] that *moral* facts are natural phenomena that emerge through *reason* alone" (1973a, 121). One notes the contrast here with Weber's summary dismissal of the very possibility of a "science of morality": "an empirical science," Weber says, "cannot tell anyone what he *should* do, but rather what he can do—and under certain circumstances—what he wishes to do"; "*the creation of . . . generally valid ultimate value-judgments cannot be . . . the task of any empirical science*" (1949, 54, italics changed, 57; see also 52).

## Classroom and Society as Intergenerational Conduits of Morality

The school classroom group, Durkheim says, "is a small society . . . [with] its own morality, [and] discipline is this morality" (1973a, 148–149), except that it "is a group of young people of the same age and generation. Society, on the contrary, comprises a *plurality of generations* superimposed on each other and connected with each other. . . . Without this feeling of *the bond joining generation to generation* . . . social solidarity would be singularly precarious. . . . [Therefore, the child] should be made aware of the legacy of those who preceded him" (1973a, 246–47), and, we would add, that goes both ways.

"A [school] class without discipline," then, "is like a mob. . . . But, on the other hand, it is not necessary that regulation should go to the point of the most detailed minutiae [such a society would have what *Suicide* would call a "fatalistic" culture structure]. It is indispensable that there be rules; it is unfortunate if *everything* is regulated. [Children, however, need] to sense a law beyond them which constrains and sustains them" (1973a, 515, 152). "Since it is through the teacher that [this law is] revealed to the child, everything depends on [the teacher; and the teacher's success] is entirely brought about through the teacher's respect for [the teacher's] role" (1973a, 154, 155)—analogous to Weber's description of the Lutheran idea of one's inwardly charismatic "calling."

At the same time, however, Durkheim tells us that "it is precisely groups of young persons . . . like those constituting the social system of the school, which have enabled the formation of societies larger than the family. . . . Because of [the] gathering of the young into special groups, determined by age and not by blood, extrafamilial societies have been able to come into being and perpetuate themselves" (1973a, 231–232).

We summarize these ideas in figure 2.4 and add to them a retitling of *Moral Education* as *The Division of Labor, Part 4: A Forecast of, and Preparation for, the Future Moral Education of Children Which Will Support Human Societal Self-Maintenance*. Note that this retitling makes explicit Durkheim's implication that the behavior of individuals, when controlled by social facts, feeds back to maintain those social facts.

\*

By way of summarizing this chapter, we first bring together our retitlings of Durkheim's four main substantive works. We claim that these works constitute a single theory that we would integrate under the general title *The Division of Labor in Society*. We subtitle part 1 of this theory "Social Structural and Culture Structural Mechanisms of Human Societal Self-Maintenance, and Some Possible Abnormalities Therein." We subtitle part 2 "The Suicide Rate, Empirical Indicator of Quantitative Abnor-

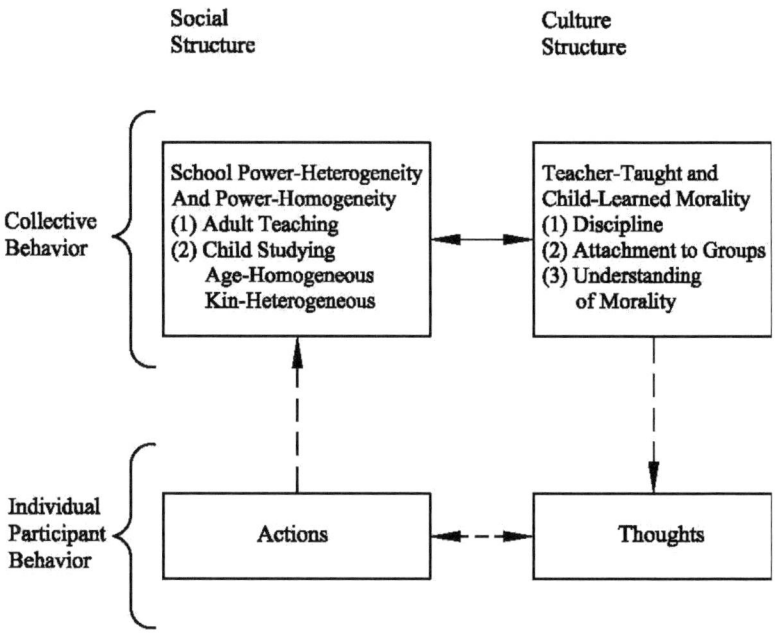

Figure 2.4. Durkheim's *Moral Education*

malities in the Social Structural and Culture Structural Mechanisms of Human Societal Self-Maintenance." We subtitle part 3 "The Religious Organizations as Initiating and Maintaining Simple Societies, and as Providing the Basis for Complex Human Societies." And we subtitle part 4 "A Forecast of and Preparation for the Future Moral Education of Children Which Will Support Human Societal Self-Maintenance."

Finally, let us summarize our reasons for proposing Durkheim's theory as the core of classical sociological theory—despite the many unresolved problems in that theory: (1) Durkheim's theory proposes that human sociocultural phenomena contribute substantially to their own maintenance (and implicitly therefore to the continued survival of our species), and that sociology's first explanatory task is to detail empirically the ways that that self-maintenance is achieved. (2) Durkheim's theory proposes two interacting mechanisms whereby every human society contributes to its self-maintenance—namely, social structure and culture structure. (3) Durkheim's theory proposes that the general direction of evolution in those two mechanisms is from simple unison to complex cooperation. (4) Durkheim's theory proposes four possible nonlinear quantitative abnormalities that may develop in those mechanisms in complex societies—two in social structure, and two in culture structure. (5) Durkheim's theory proposes a temporary sociocultural self-maintenance function of religious organizations in the production of early morality but forecasts that religious organizational dominance of morality will later be replaced by secular informational organizations as supports for the complex morality of complex societies.

In the next three chapters, we examine the particular supplements that Marx, Weber, and Ibn Khaldûn, respectively, make to this core sociological theory—and, implicitly, to sociological forecasts of human species survival.

# Part II

## Chapter 3

## MARX'S SUPPLEMENTARY THEORY: THE INDIVIDUAL HUMAN'S PHYSICAL (AND PSYCHICAL) BEHAVIORS

In sharp contrast with Émile Durkheim's *sociocultural self-maintenance claim* that "it is . . . in the nature of *society* itself that we must seek the explanation of social life," Karl Marx says that "the premises from which we begin.. . . are the real *individuals*, their activity and the material conditions under which they live," and that "the social structure and the State are continually evolving out of the life-process of *definite individuals*" (1969, 1:19, 24; see also 518; 1973, 265).[1] Weber seconds Marx rather than Durkheim here when he says "collectivities must be treated as solely the resultants and modes of organization of the particular acts of *individual persons*" (1978, 13; see also Popper 1961, 291).[2] Ibn Khaldûn holds the same view as Marx and Weber against Durkheim: "We say that *man* is distinguished from the other living things by certain qualities peculiar to him, namely: (1) . . . [the] ability to think . . . (2) [the] need for restraining influence and strong authority . . . (3) man's need for food to keep alive and subsist . . . [and] (4) human beings have to dwell in common and settle together in cities and hamlets" (1969, 42).

So Durkheim stands alone here in building his theory on a premise about the self-maintenance of *sociocultural phenomena* rather than on the individual participants' proactive behavior. Marx, Weber, and Ibn Khaldûn, however, rest their theories on premises about the particular species behavior of the *individual participants* in human societies and about the particular geographical nature of those participants' *habitats*.

Thus, (1) Marx claims that "The first fact to be established is the *physical* organization of [human] individuals and their consequent relation to the rest of nature" (1969, 1:20)—the latter phrase, of course, implicating habitat—(2) Weber says "the term 'social relationship' will be used to denote the behavior of a plurality of actors insofar as . . . the action of each *takes [psychical] account of that of the others and is [psychically] oriented in these terms*" (1978, 26); and (3) Ibn Khaldûn says "Civilization may be either *desert* (Bedouin) civilization as found in *outlying regions and mountains*, in hamlets *(near) pastures in waste regions*, and on the *fringes of sandy deserts*; or it may be sedentary civilization as found in cities, villages, towns, and small communities" (1969:43).

## *Economic Organizations: Primary Means of Human Societal and Species Self-Maintenance*

As we saw in chapter 2, Durkheim extends the idea of "division of labor" beyond the economic organizations of human societies to *all* the participant-organizing organizations of our societies. Marx, however, shares Adam Smith's focus on the *economic* organizations in human societies' participant-organizing institution on the ground that such organizations are the primary maintainers of human society through their production of subsistence for society's in-taken participants.[3] Thus Marx asserts that "the first premise of all human existence and, therefore, of all history . . . [is that] life involves before everything else eating and drinking, a habitation, clothing and many other things. *The first historical act is thus the production of the means to satisfy these needs*" (1969, 1:30). "Men begin to distinguish themselves from animals as soon as they begin to *produce* their means of subsistence" (1969, 1:20),[4] and "any distribution whatever of the means of *consumption* is only a consequence of the distribution of the conditions of *production*" (1969, 3:19).

Marx's central interest, however, was not—as was Smith's —in the division of *labor's productivity* of economic goods but in the fairness of the division of *rewards* for productive labor between the employer and employee classes,[5] and with these two classes' unequal influence on the political organizations of society.[6] (Chapter 4 discusses Weber's return to the matter of production efficiency, but in the *political* organizations where he says a particular kind of division of labor called "bureaucracy" evolves.)

## *A Thumbnail Sketch of Marx's Theory*

A major problem with reading Marx's theory is that he uses a terminology partly of his own invention and explicitly defines almost none of his terms (see Engels's comment at 1967, 1:4–5). The result is that much of the time readers are just guessing at Marx's meaning, and, of course, different readers may guess differently. For just this reason, we begin this chapter with a thumbnail sketch of what we believe is Marx's essential theory—even though when we quote the evidence in Marx's writings that we think supports this sketch, we run head-on into some of his biggest terminological vagaries and are forced to address them before our image can make sense.

Here, then, is our thumbnail sketch:

We imagine Marx's theory as a kind of historical play in two acts with a very short but essential intermezzo between the two acts. We entitle the play as a whole *Nonhuman Instruments of Labor: Driver of Human Sociocultural Evolution*. This title's reference to "evolution" acknowledges Darwin as a direct precursor of Marx. (Engels claims that "just as Darwin discovered the law of development of organic nature, so Marx discovered the law of development of human history" [1969, 3:162]).[7]

We entitle Act 1 of the play "Human Labor-Power Invents Nonhuman Instruments of Labor." This first act, then, is Marx's survey of human sociocultural history through its *entire past up to and including the present*. Act 2, however, is Marx's *forecast* of human sociocultural history over its *entire future*. The title of this act is the causal reverse of the first act; it is "Nonhuman Instruments of Labor Support Human Labor-Power." In short, the play expresses Marx's view of how the human species has created a sudden reversal of causal domination between human labor, on the one hand, and nonhuman instruments of labor, on the other.

The short intermezzo between the two acts represents the turn-around pylon from a many thousand year-long *past and present* period during which "living human labor-power" was causally dominant over nonhuman "instruments of labor" to what Marx forecasts will be and equally long or longer *future* causal dominance of nonhuman "instruments of labor" over "living human labor-power." The near-instantaneity of this turn-around is well expressed in the title of John Reed's 1919 [1960] journalistic account of the Russian Revolution—*Ten Days That Shook the World*—setting aside whether that particular revolution was really Marxian in its content or not.

Marx repeatedly tells us how important a change in the "instruments of labor" are to this turn-around: "*Every* change in the social order, *every* revolution in property relations is the essential result of the creation of new *productive forces*"; and "the social relations within which individuals produce, the social relations of production, change, are transformed, with the change and development of the material means of production, the *productive forces*" (1969, 1:88, 160).

There is, however, the terminological problem of how "productive forces" are related to living "human labor-power" and to nonhuman "instruments of labor." It is here that our sketch runs into difficulty with Marx's actual writing.

The first clue Marx gives us to resolving this difficulty is his claim that "*three* moments, the forces of production, the state of society, and consciousness, can and must come into contradiction with one another" (1969, 1:33–34; should we call this an instance of "trialectics"?). From this we must conclude that whatever "productive forces" *are*, they are *not* "the state of society," and they are *not* "consciousness."

The second clue appears when Marx uses the term "*instruments of production*" (he does not explicitly define these "instruments," but they certainly seem different from "*forces* of production" insofar as "instruments" implies an activating user whereas "forces" may be self-activating)[8] and distinguishes between "*natural* instruments of production and those *created by civilization*" (1969, 1:51). From this, one begins to gather that "instruments of production" are nonhuman physical *tools* (both found in nature and created in civilization) that are used by human labor-power in economic production. Another term soon appears in Marx's discussion that confirms this impression. This term is "*capital*," which Marx describes as "*accumulated labor*" where the "accumulation" occurs not physically but symbolically (that is, culture structurally) via the medium of invented and defined physical "*money*" (1969, 1:51).

Next, taking "productive forces" as including nonliving, nonhuman, "instruments of production" ("inventions," in the next quotation) along with living, human, economic division of labor ("commerce"), Marx tells us that "it depends purely on the extension of commerce whether the *productive forces* achieved in a locality, *especially inventions*, are lost for later development or not. . . . Only when commerce has become world commerce and has as its basis large-scale industry, when all nations are drawn into the competitive struggle, is the permanence of the acquired productive forces assured [!]" (1969, 1:55). Then, against the background of this mention of "large-scale industry," Marx speaks of "That labor which from the first presupposed a machine, even of the crudest sort, soon showed itself the most capable of development [into greater and greater power and complexity]" (1969, 1:56). This "productive force," namely, masses of *human labor* organized into "large-scale" or "big industry" (and equipped with mechanical, specifically steam-driven, instruments of labor), Marx says, "produced *world* history for the first time, insofar as it made all civilized nations . . . dependent for the satisfaction of their wants on the whole world, thus destroying the natural exclusiveness of separate nations. . . . [Its first premise] was the *automatic system*" (1969, 1:61)—and by "automatic system," Marx clearly has in mind *machine* automaticity.

So when Marx tells us that "*every* change in the social order, *every* revolution in property relations is the essential result of the creation of new *productive forces*," he includes two things in "productive forces": *the specializing division of living human labor-power*, and *equally specialized nonliving, nonhuman, machine instruments of production*.

It also should be noted that Marx imposes no time reference in this statement; he is speaking of the past in general and present and the future in general all in a single claim. He is saying that human society *always* evolves according to the human invention of (1) new ways of organizing living human labor-power (the "division of labor") and (2) new ways of organizing nonliving, nonhuman, "instruments of labor." His great forecast, moreover, is that such nonhuman machines will increasingly *replace* human labor-power in economic production.

One further problem needs to be answered before that replacement can occur, however. That problem is: who (or what) shall *plan, direct, and evaluate* the operation of the new instruments of production, and who (or what) shall *implement* those plans, directions, and evaluations? What, in short, will be the *new "property relations"* that derive from these new "instruments of production"?

To answer this question, let us back up to a moment just before the curtain falls on Act 1. The kind of "world history" that "big industry" has created depends on a particular kind of "division of labor"—one between specialists in *mental* work and specialists in *physical* work. There are, then, two socioeconomic classes composed of *mentally* working *employers*, on the one hand, and *physically* working *employees*, on the other. Thus, "Division of labor," Marx says, "only becomes truly such when a division of material and mental labor appears" (1969, 1:33)—and he does not tell us why "*only*" then. The specialist in "mental" labor plans, directs, and evaluates the labor-process while the specialist in "material" labor physically implements those plans, directions, and evaluations.

The employing specialist, however, soon discovers that his specialty gives him unforeseen opportunities to extort an increasingly disproportionate amount of production-rewards out of what Marx believes rightfully belongs to the implementer's share of rewards. Because that increasingly ravenous skim-off is forcefully supported by the armed (police and military) political organizations who have been secretly bought and paid for by rich employers, Marx argues that there is one and only one escape—namely, economic and political overthrow of the entire employer class by the armed employee class. Only then, Marx implies, can Act 2 raise its curtain on what he forecasts will be the endlessly idyllic future of all humankind.

But there are more problems in that overthrow than where the revolutionaries' weapons can come from.

Marx says "each new class which puts itself in the place of one ruling before it, is compelled [by conditions laid down, implicitly, by the ruling coalition that it wishes to form] . . . to represent its interest as the common interest of all the members of the society, that is . . . it has to give its ideas the form of universality, and represent them as the only rational, universally valid ones. . . . Its victory . . . benefits also many individuals of the other classes which are not winning a dominant position [but it] puts these individuals in a position to raise themselves into the ruling class" (1969, 1:48–49).

With the succession of class overthrows in past and present history, then, Marx says, there evolves an irreversible, long-term, periodic, accumulation: "Every new class . . . achieves its hegemony only on a broader basis than that of the class ruling previously, whereas the opposition of the non-ruling class against the new ruling class later develops all the more sharply and profoundly. Both these things determine the fact that the struggle to be waged against this new ruling class, in its turn, aims at a more decided and radical negation of the previous conditions of society than could all previous classes which sought to rule" (1969, 1:49). Especially in envisioning such a broadening basis of class hegemony, Marx forecasts his favored resolution of "the history of class struggles" which is that "the history of all hitherto existing society" (1969, 1:108) is an escalator that eventually includes *all* human individuals.

The culmination he forecasts to that escalation, then, is that the proletarian class revolution will be the *final* class revolution of human sociocultural history—the revolution that will not merely establish the proletariat as the *new* ruling class but will *abolish all classes*, rulers and ruled, and with them the whole division of labor, in all fields, forever. Once that final intermezzo is over, the curtain can rise on Act 2:

> the means [of human labor will now culminate in] an automatic system of *machinery* . . . set in motion by an automaton, a moving power that moves itself; this automaton consisting of numerous mechanical and intellectual organs, so that the workers themselves are cast merely as its conscious linkages. . . . Labor no longer appears so much to be included within the production process; rather, the human being comes to relate more as watchmen and regulator to the production process itself. . . . The free development of individualities . . . [through] the general reduction of the necessary labor of society to a minimum, which then corresponds to the artistic, scientific etc. development of the individuals in the time set free, and with the means created, for all of them [then follows]. (1973, 692, 693, 695, 705, 706)

The mechanical "automaton" that Marx mentions here (for which the brother of Karel Čapek, the Czech playwright author of "Rossum's Universal Robots," coined the word "robot") will then last, forever, with never a single complaint against it because robots are nonhuman machines that will produce all the *physical* things that humans need, leaving humans to do all the *psychical* things that were once reserved for the employing directors of the labor-process. In other words, Marx claims, *up to the present* "[human] life [has not been] determined by consciousness" (1969, 1:25) but by physical actions equipped with elementary physical instruments. In *future* human history, however, life will be determined by human consciousness because, he says, "consciousness [that is, pure science and applied science, engineering, consciousness] is something the world *must* acquire, like it or not" (1978, 15). Marx, in a word, is an evolutionary materialist when referring to our species' past and present but a utopian idealist when referring to its future.[9]

Thus ends our thumbnail sketch of Marx's theory.

Let us now try to trace out some of the principal details of Act 1. We begin with figure 3.1.

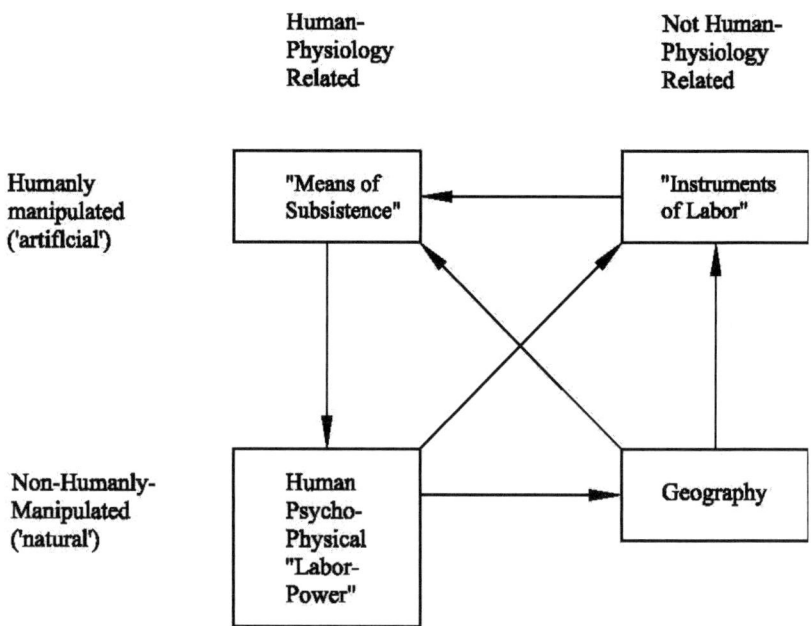

Figure 3.1. Marx's Pre-Class Division of Labor Labor-Process

## The Human Labor-Process Produces Humans' Means of Subsistence

Human economic production, Marx argues, has been carried out since early prehistoric times by the living human "labor-process," wherein "*man's* activity, with the *help* of the instruments of labor, effects [a physical] alteration, [psychically] designed from the commencement, in the material worked upon" (1967, 1:180; see also 46, 178, 181; 1922, 141, 143; 1988, 72). In our judgment, this generic "labor-process" represents the intersection of the two more abstract dimensions shown in figure 3.1. The vertical dimension distinguishes what we may call the cosmically evolved, "natural," factors from humanly constructed, "artificial" factors (Marx calls them "created by civilization," but we know now that hominid-made stone tools antedate human civilization by at least two million years).

One of the "natural" factors is genotypical of Homo sapiens ("labor-power"), and the other is the surface of our planet ("geography")—the "material" on which that "labor-power" is practiced. One of the "artificial" factors is humanly cultivated, bred, and harvested "means of human subsistence" (oxygen, water, food, clothing, shelter, medications), and the other is made up of humanly invented and constructed "instruments of human labor." The causal arrows in figure 3.1 summarize Marx's hypotheses that human labor-power (lower left) acts on geographical factors (lower right) to produce from them tools for labor's use (upper right); labor-power then acts with those tools on other geographical factors to produce means of human subsistence (upper left); the consumption of those means energizes human labor-power (lower left again) for its next action on geographical factors (lower right again)—and so on, cycle after cycle, out of humankind's deep past to the present.

## The Generic Labor-Process and the Specific Modes of Production

When Marx refers, generically, to the whole process just outlined, he uses the term "labor-process," but he tells us that that process should be considered *"independently of the particular form it assumes under given social conditions"* (1967, 1:177). This "independence" seems to us the reason (Marx himself does not explain why), when referring to some one of those changeable "particular" forms, Marx speaks of it as a "mode of [economic] production" rather than as a "labor-process":[10] *"With the acquisition of new productive facilities, men change their mode of production* and with the mode of production all the economic relations which are required by this particular mode of production" (1969, 1:519); and when he refers to the *"capitalist mode of production"* (1969, 3:19; see also 1967, 3:814–815) rather than the capitalist "labor-process"; and when, with narrower focus within capitalism, he claims that "in modern industry [revolution] begins with the [invention and introduction of] instruments of labor" (1967, 1:371).[11]

In short, the concepts "mode of production" and "labor-process" seem to refer to the *same* phenomena in Marx's theory, but the first term acknowledges that these phenomena *evolve* from one particular form or "mode" to another, while the second term ignores that *evolution* while emphasizing the *constancy* of human "labor" in it so far in human history.

## Two Meanings of "Capital"

Whether discussing the generic "labor-process" or one of its particular historical "modes of production," Marx usually distinguishes between the human genotypical *"labor-power"* that does the work (see 1969, 1:159), and the geographic and technological materials on which, and with which, that work is done. He classifies the latter materials together as *"capital"*—which, at one point, he specifies as comprising "raw materials, instruments of labor and means of subsistence of all kinds, which are utilized in order to produce new raw materials, new instruments of labor and new means of subsistence. All these *component parts of capital are creations of labor, products of labor"* (1969, 1:159). This clearly indicates that "capital" is not itself *living human labor*; "capital" is the nonhuman *"creations of labor, products* of labor," which can be used in further production.[12] However, immediately after making that point, Marx briefly warns us that "so say the economists" (1969, 1:159)—signaling that he himself would say something different.

To convey what we believe is a fair picture of what Marx himself would say, let us pause a moment to consider why he entitles his main work *Capital*. Why not "labor-power," "the proletariat," "class struggle," or, indeed, anything whose referent is more directly *human sociocultural* than *"capital"*?

Marx tells us that "a cotton-spinning jenny is a *machine* for spinning cotton. It *becomes capital only in certain [sociocultural] relations"* (1969, 1:159). Now, Marx does not mean the jenny magically *stops being a machine when it becomes capital*—any more than a printed piece of *paper* stops being paper when it is used as *money*. Marx means that when the jenny is used in the sociocultural relations called "capitalism" it becomes classifiable with all the other nonsociocultural, nonhuman things that are used by "labor-power" in capitalism—namely, "capital." But then he tells us that "capital" is *not only* "instruments of labor": "Capital *also is a social relation of production"* (1969, 1:160).

Reading that declaration, one seems compelled to ask how a nonhuman, nonliving, *machine* can be "also a [*living human*] social relation." Marx himself, indeed, does not seem comfortable arguing that it can be both—as evidenced by his arguing, not logically but rhetorically: "Are not the means of subsistence, the instruments of labor, the raw materials of which capital consists, produced and accumulated under given social conditions, in definite social relations? . . . And is it not just this definite social character which *turns the products serving for new production into capital*?" (1969, 1:160).[13]

No matter how one answers this question, however, one would still ask how the transformation that Marx indicates would also transform "*the [nonhuman] raw materials of which capital consists*" into a *human social relation.*

But Marx's argument does not need "capital to *become* a social relation of production;" it only needs the new kind of automatic, robotic, capital toward which the engineering of his own, and more so, our time, appears to be evolving to *impact causally* on human social relations, under not only human but humane planning, direction, and evaluation. With that impact and its foreseeably increasing transformation of worktime into avocational time, Marx (and at this point we would call him a science-fiction writer) says, "nobody [will have] one exclusive sphere of activity but each can become accomplished in any branch he wishes, [for] society regulates the general production and thus makes it possible for me to do one thing to-day and another to-morrow, to hunt in the morning, fish in the afternoon, rear cattle in the evening, criticize after dinner, just as I have a mind, without ever becoming hunter, fisherman, shepherd or critic" (1947, 22).[14] Capital, not class revolution, has finally destroyed the division of labor between humans as thinkers and humans as doers; Marxian class-*based* human history has finally been made class-*less*.

## The Employer versus Employee Division of Labor in Economic Organizations

The collective division of human labor, Marx says, became the main theme of human history up to the present because: "[A] single man cannot operate upon Nature without calling his own muscles into play under control of his own brain. As in the natural body head and hand wait upon each other, so *the labor-process unites the labor of the hand with that of the head. Later on [these two labors] part company and even become deadly foes"* (1967, 1:508). As a result of that parting, at first *"the history of all [subsequent] society is the history of class struggles"* (1969, 1:108) between a mentally planning, directing, evaluating employer class and a materially implementing employee class. But, after the introduction of robots (as our thumbnail sketch has indicated), both the employer and the employee classes will disappear and all humans will take over what used to be the employer class's economic functions.

The factor that centuries ago initiated the employer-employee division of labor was Malthusian population growth and its concentration in particular geographic locations. Then, Marx says, in those locations, combined labor was invented and "all combined labor on a large scale *requires*, more or less, a directing [and therefore, we would add, a planning and evaluating] authority, in order to secure the harmonious working of the individual activities. . . . A single violin player is his own conductor, an orchestra *requires* a separate one" (1967, 1:330–331). (This is a deterministic claim with which several chamber orchestras of our own times would disagree, and regarding which

Mahler, the composer-conductor, is said to have remarked that "a conductor is only a necessary evil.")

Marx argues, then, that when a human population grows in a given locality, typically the population does not risk dying out (as Malthus thought it would, from lack of subsistence), nor does part of it migrate out (as Darwin thought it would, in search of more subsistence and less competition). Instead, Smith, Marx, and Durkheim all say the entire population stays put and develops an internal, social structurally interdependent, economic division of labor between directors and implementers that is capable of producing more subsistence than could the same participants, in the same habitat, without it.

Marx, however, does not argue (as Durkheim does) that the respective specialists develop a shared "organic solidarity" whereby the expanded subsistence would be distributed in a way agreed upon by everyone as morally "fair." Instead, Marx forecasts "*an antinomy, right against right, both equally bearing the seal of the law of exchanges and between equal rights force decides*" (1967, 1:235). As a result, he says, "the history of all hitherto existing society is the history of class *struggles*"—not class cooperations.[15]

## *Employers Extort Their Profit from Employees' Labor-Power as "Surplus-Labor"*

To his claim that "the restless never-ending process of *profit-making alone* is what [the capitalist] aims at," Marx adds his crucial definition that "profit consists [in] . . . *the excess of the total labor embodied in the commodity over the paid labor embodied in it*" (1967, 3:42; see also 197; 1:176). From this assertion of a single deterministic source of profit, Marx draws his conclusion that "the directing motive, the end and aim of capitalist production is [therefore] to . . . *exploit labor-power to the greatest possible extent*" (1967, 1:331).

Note that this argument removes *profit-making* from the directors' aim, redefining their aim as winning an *interpersonal and inter-class conflict* (i.e., to "*exploit labor-power*" to the greatest possible extent"—making profit-making a side issue insofar as exploiting labor-power might well, by itself alone, not guarantee any profit at all).

Marx, however, proposes the existence of a perfect correlation between labor-power exploitation and profit-making when he tells us that "The capitalist's profit is derived from the fact that [the capitalist] has something to sell for which he has paid *nothing*" (1967, 3:42)—note: paid not less than its value but "*nothing*"—and that "something" for which "nothing" is paid is "*surplus-labor.*" "Surplus-labor," then, is a kick-back pure and simple; it is labor *extorted* by the employer from the employee in return for the employee's being allowed to hold the job at all.[16] Marx dubs the employer's interest in extortion a "*werewolf hunger for surplus-labor*" (1967, 1:265)—a hunger, note again, not for "profit," which may come from many sources, but for "surplus-*labor*" which comes only from human laborers.

Indeed, Marx seems to have considered the possibility of many alternative, and contributing, sources of employers' profits (see 1967, 3:32, 35; cf. 1:156–166; 3:37–40), so the question arises: Why would Marx settle on the idea that "surplus-*labor*" is the capitalist's *one and only* source of profit? Why wouldn't he simply claim (as did Ibn Khaldûn more than four hundred years before), "Buy cheap and sell dear. There is commerce for you" (1969, 310), which means that in order to make a profit the employer must sell the firm's product at a *total* selling price higher than its *total* production price (*including, but not limited to*, the price of labor)?

## Employer–Employee Division of Labor and Modern Class Conflict

In their "were-wolf hunger for surplus-labor," employers devote "the *whole* of [their work-time] . . . to the appropriation and therefore *control of the labor* and to the selling of the products of this labor" (1967, 1:308; see also 169, 519, 564)—for "the restless never-ending process of *profit-making alone* [which, as we saw above, he argues comes *only* from the exploitation of "surplus-labor"] is what [employers aim] at" (1967, 1:152–153). Marx offers no explanation of how this singleminded competitiveness got started except to assert, vaguely and neither logically nor causally, that "a certain stage of capitalist production . . . "*necessitates*" it (1967, 1:308).

Marx does note, however, that in the historically original planning-direction-evaluation of "combined labor," the director specialists sought much broader goals than the exploitation of "surplus-labor" alone—namely, taking "good care that the work is done in a proper manner, and that the means of production are used with intelligence, so that there is no unnecessary waste of raw material, and no wear and tear of the implements beyond what is necessarily caused by the work" (1967, 1:184–185; see also Veblen 1979, 1–46). The emergent class competitiveness of employers in planning the exploitation of "surplus-labor," however, leads to their narrowing of employees down to "the habit of doing only one thing . . . while [their] connection with the whole mechanism [of the firm] compels [them] to work with the regularity of the parts of a machine" (1967, 1:349). Employees are also forced (because they own nothing else with which to bargain for their subsistence) systematically to bargain away all of their innately human "free, conscious activity" (see 1967, 1:153), and thereby to relinquish their personal *self*-direction.

Marx argues that not only do employers force their employees to become more and more *like* machines, but employers *substitute* more and more real machines for human workers. Soon, "it is the machine which possesses skill and strength in place of the worker, is itself the virtuoso, with a soul of its own in the mechanical laws acting through it. . . . The worker's activity, reduced to a mere abstraction of well-rounded human activity, is determined and regulated on all sides by the movement of the machinery, and not the opposite" (1973, 693; see Erickson 1986, 1–8). Moreover, although machinery can certainly be used "for *shortening* the working-time required in the production of a commodity, it becomes, in the hands of capital the most powerful means . . . for *lengthening* the working-day beyond all bounds set by human nature" and for extending that long work-day to "women and children" (1967, 1:403).

Figure 3.2 summarizes Marx's hypotheses concerning this intensifying exploitation by employers of their employees' labor-power.

## *Employee Revolution in the Political Organizations*

Marx argues that because of their monopoly of the legitimate means of physical force and violence as means of societal organization, the political organizations (parties, legislatures, executives, courts, soldiers, and police officers) are the final arbiters in case of dissensus and conflict among economic (or any other societal) organizations. Only a *revolution* in those *political* organizations using superior means of force and violence (whose source, for the rebel employees, Marx does not explain), then, can achieve abolition of the politically defended exploitation by capitalists of "labor-power to the greatest possible ex-

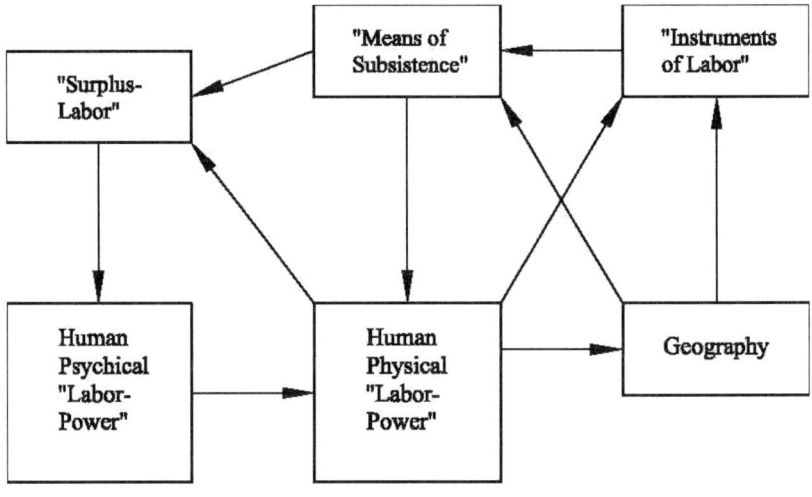

Figure 3.2. Marx's Class Division of Labor Labor-Process

tent." To this, Marx adds that "revolution is necessary [too] . . . because the class overthrowing it can only in a revolution succeed in ridding itself of all the muck of ages and become fitted to found society anew" (1947, 69). Marx does not say how or why a revolution can accomplish the revolutionaries' fitness to rule society (Fanon offers an explanation for this—see 1968, 73–95).

Marx, however, does, as a dialectician, consider that every coin may have two sides and that the capitalism coin may have done as much good as bad for the survival of the human species. Indeed, he cites six such species-serving benefits that capitalism has brought about at the cost of working-class misery—as follows.

## 1. Employers Advance the Productive Forces in Spite of Overproduction and Underconsumption Crises

While Marx condemns capitalists for heartlessly extorting more and more "surplus-labor," he also congratulates the same capitalists for having created "more massive and more colossal productive forces than have all the preceding generations together. Subjection of Nature's forces to man, machinery, application of chemistry to industry and agriculture, steam-navigation, railways, electric telegraphs, clearing of whole continents for civilization, canalization of rivers, whole populations conjured out of the ground" (1969, 1:113; cf. 159, 113).

The development of these "colossal productive forces," however, has, until now, been held back by a powerful drag: "At a certain stage of their development, the material productive forces of society come into conflict with the existing *relations of production*, or—what is but a legal expression for the same thing—*with the property relations* [between employers and employees] within which they have been at work hitherto. From forms of development of the productive forces these relations turn into their fetters" (1969, 1:503–504). "For many a decade past the history of industry and commerce is but the history of the revolt of modern productive forces [essentially, machinery] against the property relations that are the conditions for the existence of the bourgeoisie and of its rule" (1969, 1:113).[17]

This "conflict" between the "productive forces" and "property relations" takes two forms. The first form involves some employers *not using* machinery because that use would reduce the employers' profit (see 1967, 1:463–464). The second form involves other employers *using* machinery because that use puts "exceptional" profits into their pockets and less into employees' pockets. But "exceptional" profit "whets [these capitalists'] appetite for *more* profit" (1967, 1:406), and that rising "werewolf" hunger fosters swings between over- and underproduction (driven, presumably, by employers alternating between overprediction and underprediction of their future profits) and alternating, consequently, between the overemployment and underemployment of employees from whose labor those profits can be extorted (see 1967, 1:310–311, 430–437, 484–485).

As a result, "the life of modern industry becomes a series of periods of moderate activity, prosperity, over-production, crisis and stagnation" (1967, 1:453). In each "crisis" period, "suddenly . . . it appears as if a famine, a universal war of devastation has cut off the supply of every means of subsistence; industry and commerce seem to be destroyed. . . . The productive forces at the disposal of society no longer tend to further the conditions of bourgeois property; on the contrary, they have become too powerful for these conditions. . . . The conditions of bourgeois society are too narrow to comprise the wealth created by them" (1969, 1:114).

Through such booms and busts and their impacts on the workers' subsistence, together with capitalists' self-defeating efforts to control the crises while retaining the old property relations, Marx concludes, "not only has the bourgeoisie forged the weapons that bring death to itself; it has also called into existence the men who are to wield those weapons—the modern working class—the proletarians" (1969, 1:114). And after the proletarians wield those weapons successfully against governmental military and police forces, the terminated capitalist society will be supplanted (analogous to species extinction in Darwin's theory, where "old forms [are] supplanted by new and improved forms of life" [1968, 343]) by a "new and improved" human society where "the *productive forces* developing in the womb of bourgeois society create the material conditions for the solution of [the] antagonism [between the productive forces and property relations]" (1969, 1:504) by creating *new, species-beneficent, property relations* that complement rather than oppose the new productive forces.

## 2. Employers Globalize Economic Organizations

Throughout the time that the productive forces are advancing (in spite of short-term rises and falls in the business cycle), capitalism is globally consolidating its hitherto separate national economies into single, ultimately global, entities. Thus, "modern industry has converted the little workshop of the patriarchal master into the great factory of the industrial capitalist. Masses of laborers, crowded into the factory, are organized like soldiers" (1969, 1:115; see also 1967, 1:627–628)—and that crowding generates a proletarian culture structure. "With the development of industry the proletariat not only increases in number; it becomes concentrated in greater masses, its [social structural] strength grows, and it [culture structurally] feels that strength more. . . . This union is helped on by the improved means of communication that are created by modern industry and that place the workers of different localities in contact with one another [welding them]. . . . into one national struggle between classes" (1969, 1:116; see also Durkheim 1965, 245–247).

Beyond these national struggles, Marx says, there emerges one global struggle. "*Big industry . . . produced world history* for the first time, insofar as it made all civilized nations and every individual member of them dependent for the satisfaction of their wants on the whole world, thus destroying the former natural exclusiveness of separate nations" (1969, 1:61).[18]

## 3. Employers Consolidate Multiple Classes into Only Two Classes Globally

Not only does capitalism consolidate national economic organizations, it also consolidates the different classes within nations: "Our epoch, the epoch of the bourgeoisie . . . possesses this distinctive feature: it has *simplified* the class antagonisms: Society as a whole is more and more splitting up into *two* great hostile camps, into *two* great classes directly facing each other: Bourgeoisie and Proletariat" (1969, 1:109). The bourgeoisie has achieved this consolidation largely by closing avenues of upward mobility while opening avenues of downward mobility. The result is that "the contradiction between the individuality of each separate proletarian and . . . the condition of life forced upon him, becomes evident to him himself, for he is sacrificed from youth upwards and within his own class, [he] has no chance of arriving at the conditions which would place him in the other class"—no chance, that is, except by collective violent revolution: "In order, therefore, to assert themselves *as individuals*, [the proletarians eventually realize that they, collectively,] *must overthrow* the state" (1947, 78).

By everywhere reducing the combatants to just two, and everywhere the same two, the bourgeoisie sets the stage for two worldwide alternatives, "either . . . a revolutionary reconstitution of society at large, or . . . the common ruin of the contending classes" (1969, 1:109).

## 4. Employers Clarify Class-Based Culture Structures and Their Interrelations Globally

At the same time, capitalism also destroys many culture structural delusions held by the bourgeoisie as well as the proletariat:

"It has drowned the most heavenly ecstasies of religious fervor, of chivalrous enthusiasm, of philistine sentimentalism, in the icy water of egotistical calculation. It has resolved personal worth into exchange value, and in place of the numberless indefeasible chartered freedoms, has set up that single unconscionable freedom—Free Trade. In one word, for exploitation, veiled by religious and political [psychical] illusions, it has substituted naked, shameless, direct, brutal [physical] exploitation" (1969, 1:111), which can now, Marx says, be seen for the monster it is.

## 5. Employers Drive Employees to Destroy Old Political Organizations and Construct New Ones

Viewing the *political* organizations as arenas to which contending sides in the other participant-organizing organizations (especially the economic ones) resort for final adjudication of their disputes by the application of police and military force, Marx argues that "all struggles within the State, the struggle between democracy, aristocracy, and monarchy, the struggle for the franchise, etc., etc., are merely the illusory forms in which the real struggles of the different classes are fought out among one another. . . . [Therefore,] every class which is struggling for mastery . . . must first conquer for itself *political power* in order to represent its interest in turn as the general interest" (1947, 23).

After the proletariat wins political power for itself, Marx says, it "will use its *political* supremacy to forcefully wrest, by degrees, all capital from the bourgeoisie, to centralize all instruments of production in the hands of the State, i.e., of the proletariat organized as the ruling class; and to increase the total of productive forces as rapidly as possible" (1969, 1:126; see also 1969, 3:151). Engels, indeed, argues that political organizations will eventually utterly *disappear* from human societies because such organizations are merely manifestations of the underlying *economic class struggle* and they will disappear with a successful proletarian revolution: "State interference in social relations becomes, in one domain after another, superfluous, and then dies out of itself; the government of persons is replaced by the administration of things, and by the conduct of processes of production" (1969, 3:147).

## 6. Employers Influence Applied Scientific Information Organizations to Produce New Productive Forces and New Property Relations Globally

While all the above bourgeoisie-sponsored processes are going on, to Marx the single most important process—namely, the advance of the *engineering* side of the scientific informational organizations—is also proceeding: "the productiveness of labor . . . develops continually with the uninterrupted advance of science and technology . . . more efficient and (considering their increased efficiency) cheaper machines, tools, apparatus, etc., replace the old" (1967, 1:605). And Engels, too, tells us that "*division into classes . . . was based upon the insufficiency of production. It will be swept away [not by social revolution, but] by the complete development of modern productive forces*" (1969, 3:148).

"*The great historic quality of capital* [it is not clear whether he means capital or capitalism here]," Marx concludes, "*is to create. . . [the conditions] where labor in which a human being does what a thing [a nonliving, nonhuman, machine] could do has ceased*"(1973, 325).[19]

And with that pronouncement, we arrive at figure 3.3—representing Marx's forecast of human society after the prole-

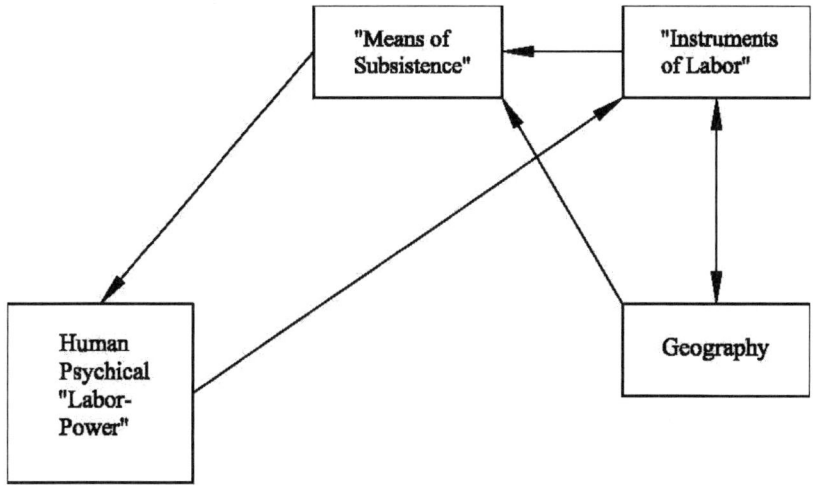

Figure 3.3. Marx's Post-Class Division of Labor Labor-Process

tarian revolution has abolished the bourgeoisie's extortion of surplus-labor from the proletariat, after bourgeois control of the political organizations has been abolished, and after engineering has turned what was living human physical labor over entirely to automatic machines.

## *Marx's Implicit Long-Term Forecast of Human Species Survival*

"At a certain point a mechanism can step into [the workers'] places," Marx says. "*What was then living worker's activity becomes the activity of the machine.* . . . [Human labor] no longer appears so much to be included within the production process; rather, the human being comes to relate more as watchman and regulator to the production process itself" (1973, 704, 705; see also 1967, 1:381). Finally, "as soon as a machine executes, without man's help, all the movements requisite to elaborate the raw material, needing only attendance from [man], we have *an automatic system of machinery, and one that is susceptible of constant improvement in its details*" (1967, 1:381).

By establishing such "an automatic system of machinery . . . set in motion by an automaton, a moving power that moves itself," then, the many-thousands-year-long *class conflict* over property relations between slave-owners and slaves, between feudal lords and serfs, and between the bourgeoisie and the proletariat can finally evolve into the mutually *cooperative* relations among all humans that Durkheim almost foresaw. At that time, all humans will be arrayed on the same planning-directing-evaluating side of the economic division of labor, while nonhuman capital is arrayed on the other, physically implementing, side—thereby permanently guaranteeing Homo sapiens' survival fitness.

We of the twenty-first century, however, must add our forecast that sooner or later all Earthly raw materials for the production of such automatic machinery and for the production of human subsistence must be physically exhausted, and Marx's proposed extension of the human species' Earthly life-span must then cease to hold. At that point, our descendants will have to move on to some more hospitable planet if that life-span is to be extended.

## Chapter 4

## WEBER'S SUPPLEMENTARY THEORY: THE INDIVIDUAL HUMAN'S PSYCHICAL (AND PHYSICAL) BEHAVIORS

In this chapter, after examining Weber's treatment of the human individual's *psychical* behavior characteristics—including his discussion of meaning, ten separate but logically integrable types of rationality, and charisma as one of two types of non-rationality—we acknowledge his touching briefly on the individual's *physical* behavior capabilities. We then examine Weber's study of a diffusion of culture structure from religious organizations to economic organizations of Western European societies, and that influenced the rise of capitalism there.[1]

### *Conscious Human Psychical Behavior*

Max Weber is the classical sociological theorist of *conscious* participation in human sociocultural phenomena—as Sigmund Freud is the classical theorist of *unconscious* participation. Freud tells us that "in a group, the individual is brought under conditions which allow him to throw off the repressions of *his unconscious instinctual impulses*. The apparently new characteristics which [the individual] then displays are in fact the manifestations of this unconscious, in which all that is evil in the human mind is contained as a predisposition" (1959, 6).[2]

Weber, by contrast, does not even mention unconscious psychical processes; instead, he focuses entirely on *conscious* psychical behavior: we humans, he says, "are *cultural* beings, endowed with the capacity and the *will* to take a *deliberate* attitude towards the world and to lend it significance. Whatever this significance may be, it will lead us to judge certain phenomena of human existence in its light and to respond to them as being . . . *meaningful*" (1949, 81). He tells us that "there is *nothing in . . . things themselves* to set some of them apart as alone meriting attention" (1949, 78) so that only the variable *attribution*, by humans, of anthropocentric subjective meaning to people and other things makes some of them *seem* more important than others.

The "meaning" we attribute to things, he says, expresses our estimation of their relation to "*human* action in the role *either of means or of end*; a relation of which the actor or actors can be said to have been *aware* and to which their action has been oriented" (1978, 7). "Meaning," then, to Weber, is always *human*-centered and oriented to achieving *humanly* defined ends.[3]

A given means-end pair constitutes a human "*motive*" to Weber—such that "we understand in terms of *motive* the meaning an actor attaches to [a physical behavior] in that we understand *what [end-in-view] makes him do this [as means to that end] at precisely this moment and in these circumstances*," and that a "correct causal interpretation of a concrete course of action is arrived at when the *overt* [physical] action and the [covert, psychical] *motives* [of all the participants in a collective action] have both been correctly apprehended and . . . their relation has become meaningfully comprehensible [to observers]" (1978, 8)[4]—thus overlooking, Ibn Khaldûn would remind us, the geographical and technological settings in which those motives and actions occur.

How does an individual human "actor" psychically construct a means–end coupling—that is, a "motive"? This is the question around which we shall try to organize Weber's conceptualizations of human rationality and nonrationality. We phrase our argument as though it addressed the problem of how an individual considers a *means* for a given end (for example, how to get from here to there), but it also addresses the problem of how an individual considers *ends* for a given means (for example, what to do with a given amount of money, power, honor and self-confidence, or knowledge and know-how) almost as well, but more complicatedly.

## *Weberian Rationality: An Inferred Generic Definition*

We begin by noting Weber's distinction between constructing motives in *rational* ways and what we shall call *nonrational* ways (unfortunately, Weber himself gives the latter ways no generic name—nor does he give us an explicit definition of rationality or of nonrationality—so we must infer what those definitions might have been had he done so). We start by inferring a Weberian definition of *rationality* (and then of nonrationality) from his more discursive descriptions.[5]

Consider two situations: (1) a subject human individual has already chosen a given end and somehow (it doesn't matter how) has in mind *only one fixed means* to that end; (2) the individual has already chosen a given end and somehow has in mind *two or more alternative means* to that end. The second situation is where Weber's idea of "rationality" arises—although he does not tell us so. That is, Weberian rationality arises whenever an individual makes *rule-bound comparisons of alternative means* to facilitate *choosing* one of them and *acting* physically on the world with it.[6]

The means being compared may be any things at all; they may seem closely related or completely unrelated; they may be proposed to the individual in any way, from any source. The rationality-defining situation exists when the individual compares, according to some consciously held rules, two or more alternatives as possible means to be chosen in pursuit of some already chosen end.

## *Different Weberian Descriptions of Rationality*

Weber seems repeatedly to *imply* the definition of rationality just given, but he never says so explicitly. He comes close when he says "rational technique is a choice of means which is consciously and systematically oriented to the experience and reflection of the actor, which consists, at the highest level of rationality, in scientific knowledge"; "rational action [is] integrated as to meaning, end, and means, and governed by principles and rules" (1978, 65, 549); and "the acting person weighs, insofar as he acts rationally . . . the various 'possible modes' of his own conduct [i.e., means] and the consequences which these could be expected to have in connection with the 'external' conditions. He does this in order to decide . . . in favor of one or another mode of action as the one appropriate to his 'goal'" (1949, 165, italics removed).

Let us set that "in order to *decide*" phrase aside and stick to the predecision comparison for a moment.

These descriptions of rationality by Weber take several things for granted that our own definition tries to bring out explicitly. First, the descriptions take for granted that the rational individual is guided by *rules*—this accounts for the importance Weber gives to the analysis of *law* as explicitly written and legally enforced rules (see 1978, 294, 312, 313). So, too, when he refers to the "transition from empirical to rational technology" (1951b, 151), Weber seems to be referring to the probably prehistoric transition from individuals' hit-or-miss comparisons to comparisons made by groups of persons according to *rules* that they accept as part of their culture structure (see 1981, 179).

Second, Weber's descriptions take for granted that the comparison of alternative means not only must be rule-bound; it must also be *consciously* so—that is, the individual must be consciously "*aware*" of and "*deliberately*" follow these rules.

Third, the descriptions take for granted that the substantive *content* of the rules (that is, what the rules tell the individual to think, feel, or do) are *irrelevant* to the definition. That is to say, such content may vary widely without disturbing the rules' rationality as long as they regulate the comparison of alternative means to a given end.

This latter stipulation is probably why Weber tells us that "we have to remind ourselves . . . that 'rationalism' may mean very different things . . . in spite of the fact that they belong inseparably together"; that "'rationalism' is a historical concept that contains within itself a world of contradictions" (1946, 293; 2002, 37; see also 1978, 655–658, 998). The only examples of that "world of contradictions" Weber gives us are when he claims that "there is . . . rationalization of mystical contemplation . . . just as much as there are rationalizations of economic life, of technique, of scientific research, of military training, of law and administration" (1958a, 26; see also 1978, 815); and that "the following methods are rational, methods of mortificatory or of magical asceticism, of contemplation in its most consistent forms. . . . In general," Weber says, "all kinds of practical ethics that are systematically and unambiguously oriented to fixed goals of salvation are 'rational'" (1946, 293–94).

What counts with Weber in determining rationality, then, is the individual's conscious reliance on rules that govern comparison of *any* kind of means toward *any* kind of end.

Now although Weber does not tell us this, the root meaning of "rational" (and of Weber's original German *rational,* and *Rationalität*) derives from *numerical calculations* (see Partridge 1959, 553, who cites *rate, ratio,* and *ration* as cognates; see also *Ration, rational,* etc., in *New Muret-Sanders Encyclopedic Dictionary of the English and German Languages*). Thus, following this definition, Weber tells us that "all *non*rational means [are] . . . practices the result of which is *not calculable*" (1978, 1172), and that "a system of economic activity will be called 'formally' rational according to the degree in which the provision for needs . . . is capable of being expressed in *numerical, calculable terms*, and is so expressed" (1978, 85). So we have a possible ambiguity: on the one hand, Weber says that "*all* kinds of practical ethics that are . . . oriented to fixed goals ... are 'rational,'" but on the other hand, he says *only* those ethics that are "capable of being expressed in *numerical, calculable terms*" are rational.

### Ten Types of Integrable Weberian Rationality

The key to resolving this ambiguity seems to be Weber's specification (quoted above) that "a system . . . will be called *formally* rational [if it] is capable of being expressed in numerical, calculable terms," for that tells us that Weber has in mind a particular *type* of rationality ("*formal* rationality"), and we must know what that type is.

Actually, our problem in understanding Weber is much thornier than that. Weber identifies ten types of procedures that he calls "rational"—namely, *Zweckrationalität, Wertration-*

*alität*, theoretical rationality, practical rationality, subjective rationality, objective rationality, low and high formal rationality, and planning and evaluating rationality. Although Weber compares certain pairs of these (for example, subjective and objective rationality), he does not compare them all together. We shall try to do that.

Our first question asks what *types of phenomena* constitute the *targeted end* that the compared means must serve?

The point of this first question is that in order to compare different means to a given *end*, that end must first be well defined. In other words, to pick out a particular *arrow* with any hope of hitting and affecting a given target with it, one must first know that *target's* materials, location, environs, size, shape, velocity, and so on. Know your targeted end is the very first means-selection directive.

In addressing this directive, Weber's first step is an easy one: He divides the universe into two jointly exhaustive categories of end-targets: the *self* of the means-comparing individual, and *everything else*. Weber's first kind of rationality, *Zweckrationalität* (literally, practical rationality), then, compares means that serve *the comparing individual her/himself as end*; and his second type, *Wertrationalität* (literally, value rationality), compares means that serve anyone and anything else—as follows.

***(1) Zweckrationalität (Self-Interest Rationality) and (2) Wertrationalität (Other-Interest Rationality).*** At first glance, Weber's definition of *Zweckrationalität* seems to reduce, nonsensically, to an infinite regress of comparisons: "Action is instrumentally rational (*zweckrational*) when the end, the means, and the secondary results are all rationally taken into account and weighed. This involves rational consideration of alternative means to the end, of the relations of the end to the secondary consequences, and finally of the relative importance of different possible ends" (1978, 26).

But by pointing out that *Zweckrationalität* involves "the relative importance of *different possible ends*" (see also 1978, 65), he implicitly commits himself to ask: what is the *ultimate* end toward which all those "*different* possible ends" may be treated as means-links in one or more causal chains that the individual expects will eventually produce that ultimate end? His answer to this question is that *personal self-interest* is the ultimate end in question: "a *uniformity* of orientation," he says, is "'determined by *self-interest*' if . . . the actors' conduct is instrumentally (*zweckrational*) oriented toward identical expectations" (1978, 29).

On that basis, it seems fair to conclude that in Weber's view, all humans have the same genotypic endowment of self-interest. Thus he says "the 'true' economic interest . . . is among the most *fundamental and universal* components of the actual course of interpersonal behavior" (1978, 601)—and "belief in 'freedom of his will' is of precious little value to the manufacturer in the competitive struggle or to the broker on the stock exchange" (1975a, 193). Such individuals, Weber implies, compare means that serve their own self-interests (*Zweckrationalität*), no matter what other beliefs they may have.

Let us, therefore, propose an English paraphrase of *Zweckrationalität* as "*instinctive self-interest rationality*," on the ground that that paraphrase is more accurate than the until-now established translation—namely, "instrumental rationality" (see 1978, 24)—because the latter translation misleads us into thinking *Wertrationalität* is *not* instrumental, when actually it *is* instrumental, but to a *different end* than one's own self-interest.

Thus, Weber says "examples of pure value-rational [*wertrational*] orientation would be the actions of persons who, re-

*gardless of possible cost to themselves*, act to put into practice their convictions of what seems to them to be required by *duty, honor, the pursuit of beauty, a religious call, 'personal loyalty,' or the importance of some 'cause' no matter in what it consists*" (1978, 25). It is the phrase "regardless of possible cost to themselves," in particular, that tells us the individual's interest in *Wertrationalität* is not the instinctive *self*-interest that dominates in *Zweckrationalität* (which centers precisely on cost to oneself), and the examples Weber provides tell us the focus of *Wertrationalitat* is one or more socioculturally *learned*, not instinctive, ends (contrast this interpretation with Bryan Wilson's view [1979, xiv, n.1]).

*Wertrationalität*, then, seems better paraphrased as "*learned non-self-interest rationality*" than as "value-rationality" (1978, 24) because the latter misleads us into thinking *Zweckrationalität* does *not* pertain to values, when actually it *does* pertain to values, specifically, to *self-interest* values.[7]

Note the weight in influencing human history that Weber assigns to the distinction between *Zweckrationalität* and *Wertrationalität* when he says, "The broad masses are occupied in the fight to secure their daily needs [*Zweckrationalität*]. . . . But in great moments, in [times] of war, their souls too become conscious of the significance of national power. Then it emerges that the national state rests on deep and elemental psychological foundations [*Wertrationalität* seems implied] . . . that it is by no means a mere 'superstructure,' the organization of the economically dominant classes" (1989b, 202, italics removed). Take that, Karl Marx!

**(3) Theoretical Rationality and (4) Practical Rationality.** The next problem is: Does the rational individual want to affect her/his *psychical understanding of*, or her/his *physical influence over*, the targeted end? This is the distinction between what

Weber calls "theoretical" and "practical" rationalities, and what we meant in chapter 3 by distinguishing between science and engineering. "'Rationalism,'" Weber says, "means one thing if we think of . . . an increasing *theoretical [understanding]* mastery of reality by means of increasingly precise and abstract concepts. Rationalism means another thing if we think of the methodical attainment of a definitely given and *practical [physical]* end by means of an increasingly precise calculation of adequate means" (1946, 293).

Both theoretical and practical rationality, then, meet our generic criterion of requiring consciously rule-guided comparisons among alternatives—but theoretical rationality compares alternative ways of *understanding* the world, whereas practical rationality compares alternative ways of *influencing* the world.

***(5) Subjective Rationality and (6) Objective Rationality.*** Weber tells us that "without the belief in the *reliability* of empirical generalizations, there could be no action based upon an estimation of the means required for an *intended* [future] result" (1975a, 132), and to this he adds that all such "reliability" extrapolations may be classified according to their "subjective" rationality and according to their "objective," "correct," or "scientific" rationality: "A subjectively 'rational' action," he says, "is not identical with a rationally 'correct' action (the latter defined as one that uses scientifically specified means). Rather, it means only that the *subjective intention of the actor* is planfully directed to the means which [that actor individually regards] as correct for a given end" (Weber 1949, 34, italics changed; see also 1981, 156)—and the individual actor, of narrow experience, is more likely to be wrong about this than right. "Magic, for example," Weber says, "has been just as systematically 'rationalized' as physics. The earliest intentionally rational therapy involved the almost complete rejection of the cure of empirical symptoms [of an ailment] by empirically tested herbs and potions in favor of the exorcism of (what was thought to be) the 'real' (magical, daemonic) cause of the ailment. Formally, it had exactly the same highly rational structure as many of the most important developments in modern therapy" (1949, 34; see also 1978, 400),[8] but its reliability was much lower.

We infer that, in these remarks, Weber has in mind two orthogonal dimensions for assessing the reliability of empirical generalizations about the effect of a given means on the targeted end. One dimension contrasts the low reliability conferred by the judgment of a *lone* individual with the much higher reliability conferred by the judgmental consensus of a *group* of individuals. The other dimension contrasts the low reliability conferred by *observationally unsupported* assertions with the much higher reliability conferred by statements based on *sensory observations*. The lowest reliability, then, goes to the lone individual who scorns sensory observations, and the highest reliability goes to the group that relies on its members' sensory observations.

Thus, Weber says, "it is one of the essential features of [a scientific] account that it aims at *intersubjectively* valid 'objective truth'"; and the "'motives' [underlying a given human action] are in principle always subject to verification on the ground of *observational* experience" (1975a, 148, 198;).[9] Consequently, Weber argues, "only an *empirical discipline* . . . [presumably, he means a *group* of persons trained rigorously to follow the same set of rules in comparing alternative hypotheses] . . . can determine whether 'technical progress' exists" (1949, 35).

*(7) Low Formal Rationality and (8) High Formal Rationality.* "The term '*formal* rationality of economic action' [designates] the extent of *quantitative calculation* or accounting

which is technically possible and which is actually applied," and "a system of economic activity will be called *'formally'* rational according to the degree in which the provision of needs . . . is capable of being expressed in *numerical, calculable* terms, and is so expressed" (cited earlier).[10]

When one notices Weber's reference here to quantitatively calculable rationality as having a *variable* "extent" and a *variable* "degree," we are reminded of Stevens's (1946) analysis of these matters—although Stevens does not mention Weber's work. Stevens posits four types of measurement scales (called "nominal," "ordinal," "interval," and "ratio") and orders them according to whether they contain a natural origin (zero-point), and whether the distances between points on their scales have unambiguous meaning. "Nominal" scales permit only the *lowest* degree of precision in measurement, whereas "ratio" scales enable the *highest* degree of precision; "ordinal" and "integral" scales have second highest and third highest degrees of precision, respectively.

A vague anticipation of such a scale of scales as Stevens proposes seems to underlie Weber's claims that "*both* calculation in kind [nominal scale] and in money [ratio scale] are *rational* techniques" (1978, 107), but that "expression in money terms yields the *highest degree* of formal calculability" (1978, 85; see also 1978, 100–107; 1975a, 121). His references to "degrees" of "formal rationality," then, seems to refer, not to some *unique* measurement process, but to what Stevens tells us is a *range* of different measurement processes (cf. Marcuse 1971, 136).

Such a *range* of "formal rationality" enables us to understand Weber's assertion that "formal rationality and substantive rationality [may be] in *conflict*" (1946, 331; see also Mommsen 1974, 69; Albrow 1990, 133). In establishing a context for this assertion, Weber says, "The more the world of the modern capitalist economy [relies on money], the less accessible it is to any imaginable relationship with a religious ethic of brotherliness. . . . [That ethic cannot regulate] the relations between the shifting holders of mortgages and the shifting debtors of the banks that issue these mortgages: for in this case, no personal bonds of any sort exist. If one nevertheless tried to do so . . . formal rationality and substantive rationality [would come into] conflict" (1946, 331).

As a result, we interpret Weber as referring, in "formal" rationality, to the *precision* of one's measurement of a means' effect on the end—where, by contrast, he uses "subjective" and "objective" rationality, to refer to that measurement's *reliability*. More specifically, then, Weber seems to be claiming not that *all* degrees of formal rationality conflict with substantive rationality, but that the *low* degree of formal rationality (characterized by what Stevens calls "nominal" and "ordinal" scales) necessitated by "substantive" rationality (see below) whose criterion is nominal "brotherliness" conflicts with the *high* degree (interval and ratio scales) of formal rationality that is present in an economy that employs impersonal and empirically tested "money" (see Parsons 1937, 35–36). Indeed, as Weber finally puts the substantive-formal issue, "substantive and formal rationality [we would say the accuracy and the precision of measurement] are . . . *largely distinct* problems" (1978, 111, italics changed)—note: not *conflicting* problems but "distinct" problems, and not *entirely* distinct, but only "largely" distinct. Weber strengthens this point with the claim that lawmaking and lawfinding "are *formally irrational* when . . . recourse is had to oracles or substitutes therefor. Lawmaking and lawfinding are *substantively irrational* . . . to the extent that decision is influenced by concrete factors of the particular case . . . rather than by general norms." Weber concludes from this that "lawmaking and lawfinding may be rational in a formal *or* a substantive way" (1978, 656)—and we believe he would also say they may be rational in *both* ways if they apply "ratio" scales *and* if their scale values are compared on the basis of collective norms that apply to both.[11]

*(9) Planning Rationality and (10) Evaluation Rationality.* All eight types of rationality discussed up to this point may be grouped together as comprising a ninth, planning, type of rationality (that is, as *before-the-act assessments* of potential means). A tenth type comprises orientations that are *after-the-act evaluations* of the employment of given means (cf. Mommsen 1974, 68; see our examination of Marx's concept of employers as planners-directors-and-evaluators in chapter 3). Thus, Weber tells us that "the concept of 'substantive rationality' . . . [applies to] certain criteria of ultimate ends, whether they be ethical, political, utilitarian, hedonistic, feudal, egalitarian, or whatever, and measures the *results* of the economic action . . . against these scales" (1978, 85–86; see also 844).

And note how, with that last sentence, Weber indicates that the *evaluation* scales employed in substantive rationality should be *the same as the planning scales* employed in the other rationalities. Such identity of preaction planning and postaction evaluation criteria is essential if the observed success or failure of a past action is to be evaluated against prior expectation and if that evaluation is to be taken into account when planning the next action. This is why the relatively constant criterion of "money"—with its higher degree of formal rationality than barter—is so indispensable to modern capitalist economic action: Weber says that an "enterprise is always faced with the question as to whether any of its parts is operating . . . unprofitably, and if so, why. . . . This can be determined with relative ease in an ex-post calculation of the relation between accounting 'costs' and 'receipts' [when both are expressed] in *money* terms. . . . But it is exceedingly difficult to do this entirely in terms of an *in-kind* calculation" (1978, 102).

In summary, then, Weber's discussion of procedures governing rational comparison may be systematized as follows. The first eight types, taken together, constitute a ninth type that governs preaction *planning*-of-means-selection (which is to say, self versus other; theoretical versus practical; subjective versus objective; low formality versus high formality). The tenth type (called "substantive") pertains to *whether a postaction evaluative measurement* as well as *a preaction planning measurement* should be made, or just the latter. If both should be made, then, presumably, the first eight types should be performed before, and the second eight types should be performed after, each means application in order to make sure the means was properly applied and that the targeted end was actually affected as desired.

## *Choosing among Alternative Means or Ends*

Now suppose all eight types of planning rationality discussed so far, and all eight types of evaluation (or "substantive") rationality, have been applied to the *comparison* of alternative means to a given end. How does the rational individual go about *choosing* one of those compared means actually to apply to that end first?

It is a striking and essential (though undeclared) part of Weber's argument that he offers no *rational* method for making choices among different end-targets, and no *rational* method for making choices among alternative means toward any given end-target after they have been compared. He simply does not tell us whether self is ultimately more rational than other, or whether subjective rationality is ultimately more rational than objective rationality in a given case; he only says they are *both* rational. Bologh, then, seems only half right when she says that "there is *no rational method for determining values* as there is for choosing among alternative means" (1984, 176; see also Giddens 1979, 42; Dahrendorf 1987, 577), for there is also no rational method, according to Weber, for determining *means*. To construct either such rational methods, he implies, one would have to be omniscient.

Weber does not leave us utterly without guides for choosing among compared means and among compared ends, however. He proposes two "ethical standards of behavior" that are relevant here, although he calls neither standard "rational."

## *Ethical Standards of Behavior*

Weber calls the contrast between these two standards an "abysmal" one (he does not tell us why he calls it this). One standard he calls "*an ethic of ultimate ends*—that is, he says, in religious terms, 'The Christian does rightly and leaves the results [presumably including side-effects and ultimate ends] with the Lord'"; the other standard he calls "*an ethic of responsibility* . . . [where] one has to give an account of the foreseeable results of one's action" (1946, 120). (Weber does not say to whom that account should be given, but one guesses he would say, at least, "oneself.") It therefore appears that an "ethic of ultimate ends" tells the individual to choose the means that is expected (either subjectively or objectively) to show the highest *effectiveness* in producing the targeted end. In other words, this "ethic" says *never mind the cost* to all other possible ends ("Damn the torpedoes"; the omniscient Lord will defend us against those torpedoes if it is ultimately Best to do so); choose whatever means promises to secure the most desired benefit to the particular end you are now pursuing ("Full speed ahead!"). An "ethic of *responsibility*," however, says choose the means with the highest *efficiency*—that is, choose the means that promises the most beneficial effect to your chosen end *at the least cost to all the other ends* you hold dear. In other words, maximize your *net* benefit.

In sum, then, Weber claims that the choice of a given means or end may be guided by a vastly life-*complicating* motto that says, "I must take responsibility for *everything* relating to the choices that I make," or by a vastly life-*simplifying* motto that says, "I *cannot possibly* be responsible for everything; I am severely limited and can only do my best." To this, Weber adds that "one cannot prescribe to anyone whether he should follow an ethic of absolute ends or an ethic of responsibility, or when the one and when the other" (1946, 127)—it is solely the individual's choice.

As indicated just above, we cannot know which of Weber's two ethics, if either, *should* be followed. But at least we can ask how each ethic *can* influence an individual's choices of means and of ends.

Before examining Weber's hypothetical answer to this question, consider figure 4.1 as our effort to systematize Weber's ten types of rationality together with his two types of ethical standards.

## *Weberian Nonrationality: An Inferred Generic Definition*

Now let us turn to Weber's discussion of nonrationality. Having told us that "both calculation in kind and in money are rational

|  | | Planning | Evaluating |
|---|---|---|---|
| What Is The Target End? | Self | Zweck-Rationalität | Substantive |
|  | Other | Wert-Rationalität | Substantive |

| What Aspect of The Targeted End Is Important? | Understanding | Theoretical | Substantive |
|---|---|---|---|
|  | Control | Practical | Substantive |

| How Is the Means' Effect on the Targeted End Measured? | Reliability { | Objective | Substantive |
|---|---|---|---|
|  |  | Subjective | Substantive |
|  | Perision | Formal | Substantive |

| Who Is Responsilble for Side-Effects of The Means on Other Phenomena? (Ethics) | God | Ultimate Ends | Substantive |
|---|---|---|---|
|  | Self | Responsibility | Substantive |

Figure 4.1. Weber's Eight Types of Rationality for Comparing "Means," Plus Two Types of "Ethics" for Choosing among "Means" or among "Ends"

techniques," Weber goes on to say that "there also exist [two] types of action which . . . *do not know calculation.* [Such] action may be *traditionally* oriented or may be *affectually* determined" (1978, 107; see also 1172). So whereas the *rational* orientations involve the individual's conscious, rule-guided, *comparison* of alternative means, what we shall call *nonrational* orientations (as indicated above, Weber himself does not give the two orientations any categoric name) do not consider such comparison because they do not permit the consideration of alternatives. In nonrationality there is neither calculation, nor comparison, nor choice—there is only *obedience* to a single rule, and that rule may have two different origins.

What joins a specific means to a specific end in nonrationality can be (1) "traditional" orientation, Weber says, which is "very often a matter of almost *automatic reaction to habitual stimuli* which guide behavior in a course which has been repeatedly followed," or (2) "affectual" orientation, which is "determined by the actor's specific affects and feeling states . . . [and] may, for instance, consist in an *uncontrolled reaction to some exceptional stimulus*" (1978, 25). In other words, it seems to be that in "traditional" nonrational orientation, a particular means is joined to a particular end by *ingrained habit*, and in "affectual" nonrational orientation, they are joined by an *instinctive predisposition* which is activated by some stimulus innately recognized as appropriate (see Lorenz 1970, 1:103–105, for discussion of "innate releasing mechanisms").[12]

Weber is arguing, then, that when the rational individual is *choosing* between compared alternatives (as in the "ethic of responsibility" and the "ethic of ultimate ends," discussed in the preceding section) what counts is not rationality but *nonrationality*—that is, whether the qualifications of one alternative elicit an "almost *automatic* reaction to habitual stimuli" (that is, it is governed by tradition) or "an "*uncontrolled* reaction to some exceptional stimulus" (that is, it is governed by affect). If either of these reactions occurs, then the choice is instantly made on its basis. Otherwise, presumably, the individual sits and ponders until such a reaction does occur. In either case, however, no one but the individual her/himself can make the choice because the individual is reacting (or waiting to react) "automatically" or "uncontrollably" to a pre-existing internal (learned, traditional; or innate, affectual) prescription.

This appears to be the sense in which the choice neither of ends nor of means can be matters of rational comparison to Weber: it is because one's choice of ends (as of means) is the province of ingrained habit or of inborn instinct and cannot be changed in the short-run. The rule here, in short, is *chacun à son goût*—although Weber never says so outright—and in the end, only the individual can bear responsibility for her/his own arbitrary taste or style in means and in ends.[13]

Weber's concept of human "motives," then, is a variable mix of rationality and nonrationality (cf. Pareto 1935, paragraphs 888–1324, 1419–1543; Coleman 1990, 14), and the *individual human sociocultural participant* is the final author of that mix and the sole captain of her/his fate.

Indeed, Weber says that "it would be very unusual to find concrete cases of action . . . which were oriented *only* in one or another of these [rational, and nonrational] ways"; that "when a civil servant appears in his office daily at a fixed time . . . [he does so] partly because disobedience would be disadvantageous to *him* [self-interest rationality] but *also* because its violation would be abhorrent to his sense of *duty* [other-interest rationality]"; that "it is even possible for the same individual to orient his actions to contradictory systems of order. . . . A person who fights a duel follows the code of [other-interest rationality] honor, but at the same time . . . he takes [self-interest rationality] account of the criminal law"; that "submission to an order is almost always determined by a *variety* of interests and by a *mixture* of adherence to [nonrational] tradition and belief in [rational] legality" (1978, 26, 31, 32, 37–38).

Weber concludes that "the action of men is not interpretable in . . . *purely rational* terms . . . not only irrational 'prejudices,' errors in thinking and factual errors but also [nonrational] 'temperament,' 'moods,' and 'affects' disturb freedom" (1975a, 125), and he almost certainly would say "the action of men is not interpretable in . . . purely *nonrational* terms" either.

## *Charisma*

In sharp contrast with Durkheim, who, as we saw in chapter 2, strives to avoid examining any proaction whatever on the part of the human individual in sociocultural phenomena, Weber tells us flatly that human action is often proactively innovative (that is, not merely reactively constrained by "social facts") and that "*the most important source of [such] innovation has been the influence of individuals,* who have experienced certain 'abnormal' states . . . and hence have been capable of exercising a special [proactive] influence on others" (1978, 321).

Weber calls the influence of such proactively innovative individuals "charisma" and claims that "in traditionalist periods, charisma is *the great revolutionary force*"; that "charisma, in its most potent forms *disrupts rational rule as well as tradition* altogether"; that "in a revolutionary and sovereign manner, charismatic domination transforms *all* values and breaks *all traditional and rational norms*"; and, in summary, "*charisma is indeed the specifically creative revolutionary force of history*" (Weber 1978, 245, 1115, 1117; cf. 1116; see also Lyman 1984,

194; Wuthnow 1987, 31; Schroeder 1992, 9).[14] According to Weber, then, the effect of charisma is to affectively *disrupt* established culture structural and social structural routines, laying those routines open to revolutionary change and reroutinization of the sort, say, that Marx says has occurred several times during small revolutionary intermezzos in the past and will occur once more during the great intermezzo of the future.

But what *is* it—what is this thing Weber calls "charisma"? There is some ambiguity in his definitions: on the one hand, he defines "charisma" as "a certain *quality of an individual personality* by virtue of which he is considered extraordinary and treated as endowed with supernatural, superhuman, or at least specifically exceptional powers or qualities. . . . How the quality in question would be ultimately judged from any ethical, aesthetic, or other such point of view is naturally entirely indifferent for purposes of identification." But to this emphasis on charisma as a proactive personal quality, Weber adds that "what is alone important is *how the individual is actually regarded* by . . . his 'followers' or 'disciples'" (1978, 241–242) (It is not clear why only the individual's "followers" should matter and not also her/his opponents and other nonfollowers.)

The first remarks mean that, to Weber, charisma belongs *objectively to its object,* but the second remark means that charisma lies in the *audience's subjective attribution*—whether or not that attribution is occasioned by some objective quality of the object. The latter seems to be the meaning to which Weber, on balance across all his sometimes contradictory comments, holds. For example, he tells us that "It is the *recognition on the part of [spectators]* which is *decisive* for the validity of the charisma . . . if the *people withdraw their recognition*, the master becomes a private person" (1978, 242, 266, 1115; also see Coleman 1990, 75).[15]

What characteristic of "the people," then, leads them to give (or withhold or withdraw) that recognition? Whatever it is, it seems very close to what Weber calls "affect," and we recall Weber's description of "*affectual*" orientation as involving spectators' "specific affects and feeling states . . . [and] may, for instance, consist in [their] *uncontrolled reaction to some exceptional stimulus*" (quoted above), and that this orientation is one of two that "*do not know calculation*" (quoted above).

Now although these statements would justify viewing charisma as a noncomparing, *nonrational* orientation, the very concept of "exceptionality" implies such *comparison*—in the sense that only comparison with stimuli already provisionally defined as *un*exceptional can define a stimulus as "exceptional." On that argument, it seems fair to say there is some *rationality* (i.e., some rule-bound comparison of alternatives) embedded in Weber's argument that an "uncontrolled reaction to some exceptional stimulus" does not involve the calculation of (formal) rationality. The same, of course, would apply to the process whereby one judges a stimulus as more cathectically *affectual* (positively or negatively) than other alternatives, and also the process whereby we judge a stimulus as more traditionally *imperative* (that is, the chosen alternative must by custom either be approached unconditionally or must be avoided unconditionally) than other alternatives.

In the end, then, both nonrational affect and some rational comparison seem implicit in Weber's reference to the charismatic "master" as presenting "some exceptional stimulus" to onlookers—as does the master who presents a "traditional" stimulus.

## Possible Objects of Charisma

What sorts of phenomena are likely to become objects of charisma attribution, according to Weber? The answer appears to be the same as Durkheim gives when he says that "a rock, a tree, a spring, a pebble, a piece of wood, a house, in a word *anything*, can be sacred" (quoted in chapter 2). That is, *anything* can become an object of charisma attribution. Weber explicitly includes "*natural objects, artifacts, animal or persons*"; bureaucratic "*office*"; "a *social institution*"; and ideas—for example, "*Reason*" itself (1978, 401, 1140, 1209)—as liable to be viewed as "charismatically endowed" (1978, 401). But let us focus on individual "persons" and ask when are persons liable to have charisma attributed to them, according to Weber.[16]

**Individual Persons as Charismatic: Erotic Love, Esthetic Pleasure, and Religiosity.** Weber, Freud, and Simmel are the only classical sociological theorists who discuss either erotic love or esthetic pleasure as human sociocultural phenomena, and Weber clearly indicates his view of them, as well as of religious devotion, as being charismatic experiences: "the *erotic* frenzy," Weber says, "stands in unison . . . with the orgiastic and charismatic form of *religiosity*," and "the creative *artist* [may experience] his work as resulting either from a charisma of 'ability' (originally magic) or from spontaneous play" (1946, 349, 341).

In suggesting that erotic love manifests an innate human capacity for attributing charisma to other humans, Weber refers to "the peculiar irrationality of the sexual act, which is ultimately and uniquely unsusceptible to rational organization" (1978, 603–604). It therefore seems fair to say that Weber regards erotic love as cathectic in its orientation, but he does not so clearly state his view of esthetic pleasure.[17]

Thus, although the "constitutive values" of art "are quite different from those obtaining in the religious and ethical domain" (1978, 608), Weber does not say what these values are—nor, surprisingly to us who come after expressionism, does he consider how esthetic values might relate to erotic values. He does, however, relate erotic values to religious values ("Originally the relation of sex and religion was very intimate. Sexual intercourse was very frequently part of magic orgiasticism or was an unintended result of orgiastic excitement"—and in "magical orgiasticism . . . every ecstacy was considered 'holy'" [1946, 343]). He also relates esthetic values to religious ones ("Religion and art are intimately related in the beginning" [1978, 607], and "magical religiosity stands in a most intimate relation to the esthetics sphere. Since its beginnings, religion has been an inexhaustible fountain of opportunities for artistic creation" [1946, 341]).

In time, however, contradictions by other aspects of culture structure with religious charisma emerged in the case of erotic as well as esthetic charisma (a three-way competition of charismas): "a certain tension between religion and sex came to the fore . . . with the temporary cultic chastity of priests . . . [and] subsequently the prophetic religions, as well as the priest-controlled life orders, have . . . regulated sexual intercourse in favor of *marriage*. The contrast of all rational regulation of life with magical orgiasticism [elsewhere, however, Weber also says that "Magic . . . has been just as systematically 'rationalized' as physics" (1949, 34)] and this has expressed "all sorts of irrational frenzies" (1946, 344; see also 1978, 603). As a result, nowadays, "the euphoria of the happy lover . . . always meets with the cool mockery of the genuinely religiously founded and the radical ethic of brotherhood" (1946, 348).

Esthetic charisma, too, was contradicted by religious charisma: "The sublimation of the religious ethic and the quest for salvation, on the one hand, and the evolution of the inherent logic of art, on the other, have tended to form an increasingly tense relation" (1946, 341). The lover "knows himself to be freed from the cold skeleton hands of rational orders. . . . This inner, earthly sensation of salvation by mature love competes in the sharpest possible way with the devotion of a supra-mundane God, with the devotion of an ethically rational order of God" (1946, 347–348).

Regarding the evolution of esthetic charisma and its relation to religious charisma, Weber says "art takes over the function of a this-worldly salvation. . . . It provides a salvation from the routines of everyday life, and especially from the increasing pressures of theoretical and practical rationalism. With this claim to a redemptory function, art begins to compete directly with salvation religion" (1946, 342, italics removed; see also 1978, 608–610).

Weber, then, sees erotic charisma, esthetic charisma, and religious charisma as affects that provide different nonrational escapes from the more rigorously demanding rationalities of everyday life (see also Shils 1987, 569).

***Geographical and Technological Objects of Charisma.*** On the charismatic potential of geographical features within which very nearly all human sociocultural phenomena have taken place so far, Weber argues that

> Jahweh . . . was originally a god of the great catastrophes of nature. His appearance is accompanied by phenomena such as earthquakes . . . volcanic phenomena . . . subterraneous . . . and heavenly fire, the desert wind from the South and South East . . . and thunder

storms. . . . flashes of lightning are his arrows. . . . For Palestine the orbit of nature catastrophes comprised also the insect, above all, the locust plague, which the South Eastern wind brought into the country. Hence the god punishes the enemies of his people with locusts and he sends swarms of locusts to confound them. He sends snakes en masse to punish his own people. (1952, 128–129)

Where Durkheim asserts categorically that "*morality* is the indispensable minimum, that which is strictly necessary, the daily bread without which societies cannot live," Weber flatly contradicts the application of that view to modern society: "on the whole," he says, "modern capitalism is . . . *emancipated from the importance of . . . ethical factors*" (1978c, 1124, 1125). "The *mechanization* of technology . . . [is] decisive for capitalism in its contemporary form" (Weber 1978c, 1128). Thus, Weber says, "the Puritan *wanted* to be a person with a vocational calling [discussed below]; we are *forced* to be [such persons]. . . . Tied to the *technical and economic conditions at the foundation of mechanical and machine production*, this cosmos today determines the style of life of all individuals born into it" (2002, 123).[18]

Considering, then, what Weber says about the possibility that human "artifacts" may become "charismatically endowed," it would appear that Weber divides Marx's reference simply to "change and development of the material means of production" into three distinct steps—namely, (1) new "material means of production" must come to be *cognitively* regarded as potentially more exceptional in producing given outcomes than the more established means; (2) that judgment must then elicit sufficient *cathectic* enthusiasm to invest in a *conative* trial of the new means and its comparison with the old means, and finally, if both these trials are passed, (3) the new means must be physically substituted for the old means in the production process.

**_Connotations of Divinity Not Required for Charisma._** Other commentators on Weber's work have linked charisma to *religion alone*, ignoring its connections (discussed above) to the erotic and esthetic—and also to the geographic, and technological spheres—of human sociocultural life. Parsons says that "charisma . . . is the quality which attaches to men and things by virtue of their relations with the '*supernatural*' " (1937, 668; cf. 1947, 75–76); Marcuse says that charisma "contains the pre-judgment that endows every form of successful personal leadership with a *religious* aura" (1971, 145); while Shils claims that "charisma . . . is the quality which is imputed to persons, actions, roles, institutions, symbols, and material objects because of their presumed connection with *'ultimate,' 'fundamental,' 'vital,' order-determining powers*" (1968, 386, see also 387); and Bradley claims that Weber held that "recognition and legitimation of [the charismatic] leader's authority [must be] based on 'sign' or proof of *divine grace*" (1987, 33).

Against all such claims, however, Weber himself asserts that charisma "derives from the surrender of the faithful [audience] to the *extraordinary and unheard-of* [event], to what is alien to all regulation and tradition and *therefore* is viewed as divine. . . . [Charisma] enforces the inner subjection [of an audience] to the unprecedented and absolutely unique and *therefore* Divine" (1978, 1115, 1117; see also 1956, 2:665, 666). Weber thus designates the "extraordinary and unheard-of," the "unprecedented and absolutely unique," as fundamental to charisma and the "divine" as one possible derivative from it (other possible derivatives, as noted above, are the erotic and the esthetic). Weber also indicates that the "extraordinary and unheard-of" need not be revered in *positive* cathexis; it may, instead, be despised in *negative* cathexis: "Persons who are externally different are simply despised irrespective of what they accomplish or what they are, or they are venerated superstitiously if they are too powerful in the long run" (1978, 385). In this way, Weber makes room for connecting the defining cognitive attribution of exceptionality to *disliking* and *avoidance* cathectic and conative responses as well as to *liking* and *attraction* responses—and also to neutral affect, "*detached*" *interest*, responses.

We argue, then, that Weber denies any *necessary* linkage between charisma and ideas about the divine, although such ideas may well be among its outcomes (see Eisenstadt 1968, xix). Indeed, Weber himself tells us that charismatic fervor may be no less deeply rooted in what an audience thinks of as frivolous, devilish, or chaotic than in what it thinks is essential, divine, or ordered—so long as that fervor attributes *cognitive exceptionality* to its object: "For present purposes," he says, "it will be necessary to treat a variety of different types as being endowed with charisma in [my] sense. . . . Value-free sociological analysis will treat all these on the same level as it does the charisma of men who are the 'greatest' heroes, prophets, and saviors according to conventional judgements. . . . In our value-free sense of the term, an ingenious pirate may be a charismatic ruler" (Weber 1978, 242, 1113; see also Gerth and Mills 1946, 52; Lindholm 1990).

## Durkheim's Concept of "Sacred" and Weber's Concept of "Charisma"

To Durkheim, it is the *gathering together of multiple individuals* that generates in each individual a sense that something "sacred" is present. In Weber's view, however, *no* social structural "gathering" of individuals is required for charisma; any *lone* individual who directly or indirectly observes (or hears talk about, or even merely imagines from whole cloth) another individual and judges that he or she is extraordinary, can be enough to instigate a person's belief that the individual in question should be "treated as endowed with supernatural, superhuman, or at least specifically exceptional powers or qualities," and that the individual, when more widely so treated, may accumulate attributions that can lead others to disrupt established sociocultural routines.

The experience of extraordinariness, then, must occur in many individuals at the same time for Durkheim—and, as Simmel neatly puts it, "the individual *feels himself* carried by the 'mood' of the mass, as if by an external force . . . [but actually] *the individual, by being carried away [and expressing that experience to others,] carries [them] away*" (1950, 35). In the case of Weber's "charisma," however, the stimulus is the presence, in any lone individual's perception (or imagination), of some object that that individual judges to be extraordinary.

"Sacredness," for Durkheim, then, is a *culture structural* concept in which proactive individual behavior plays no role of its own; for Weber, "charisma" is reducible to a proactive non-rational *individual psychical behavior* concept—which *can* become culture structural, if other individuals are recruited to that behavior.

### The Unpredictability of Charisma

Perhaps the most important thing about Weber's conceptualization of charisma attribution is that the attribution in question occurs *unpredictably*. As indicated above, literally *anything* can be regarded as charismatic, and it can become so at *any time* and at *any place*. The closest we have found Weber to saying this outright is in his brief remark that charisma *"threatens to happen everywhere"* (1978, 1120)—leaving "any time" and "to anything" unspoken but clearly implicit. He says that "in a revolutionary and sovereign manner, charismatic domination transforms *all* values and breaks *all* traditional and rational norms"; and that "the power of charisma . . . rests upon 'heroism' of an ascetic, military, judicial, magical or *whichever* kind (1978, 1115, 1116).

So it seems fair to conclude that for all the causal *systematics* that Durkheim, Marx, Ibn Khaldûn (and Malthus and Darwin)—and, indeed, Weber himself—propose are at work in human sociocultural phenomena and in the human species, Weber asserts the additional working of an intrinsically *random, unsystematic, unpredictable* causal factor in human affairs—a factor that, in the end, he tells us "is indeed *the specifically creative revolutionary force of history"* (1978, 1117).

From the standpoint of that factor, one may say that in Weber's theory, it is not God that plays dice with the world (a possibility that Einstein feared might be deduced from quantum theory); it is dice that play god with the world, and play it not only in nonrationality but at the very heart of what Weber calls "rational."

## *Human Physical Behavior*

Weber *almost* commits himself to develop an image of the human sociocultural participant's *physical* behaviors when he says that "no competent scholar would deny . . . that there is an absolutely strict distinction between all 'physiological' and all 'psychological' being" (1975a, 130; see also 1978, 4; 1981, 151; 1975b, 110), and when he claims that "it is obviously not the conventional [culture structural] *rule* of greeting that tips my hat when I meet an acquaintance. On the contrary, my [physical] *hand* does it" (1977, 108). But he does not attempt to fulfill this near-commitment.

Such as it is, then, Weber's image of the human sociocultural participant's physical behavior capabilities suffers from a lack of elementary systematics. But it suffers from two other shortcomings as well. First, his image of *physical* behaviors is almost completely dependent on the investigator's having already inferred the *psychical* behaviors that he argues must have motivated the physical behaviors in question. For example, we have already seen Weber assert that "examples of pure [psychical] value-rational *orientation* would be the [physical] *actions* of persons [etc.]."

Second, whereas Weber distinguishes between *Zweckrationalität* and *Wertrationalität* partly on the basis of whether images of the effects that the individual seeks to bring about are innate in, or learned by, that individual, he draws no similar distinction in the realm of physical behavior—such as one might draw, for example, between the innate human capacity to make a wide variety of utterances and the learned capacity to make the very particular utterances called, say, Hindi or Mandarin.

In short, Weber's definitions of physical action in general ("We shall speak of 'action' insofar as the acting individual attaches a *subjective meaning* to his behavior"), and of specifically *social* action ("Action is 'social' insofar as its *subjective meaning* takes account of the behavior of others" [1978, 4]), rule out all sociocultural behavior that is not *known* to have been guided by the acting individual's psychical attribution of meaning.

Weber persists in his meaning-requiring definitions of physical action even though he admits that "there is no guarantee at all that . . . feelings [attributed to the actor by the analyst] will correspond *in any way* to the feelings of [that actor]" (1975a, 180); and even though, by asking the question "did [the participants in a given social process] consciously ascribe *any 'meaning'* at all to the process?" (1977, 112), he tacitly acknowledges that physical processes can occur without actors consciously attributing any psychical meaning whatever to their participation in them.

Nevertheless, Weber elaborates on the notion that a man's physical "hand," not the psychical "rule" in his mind, tips his hat when he says that "our most [psychical] ideal needs are everywhere confronted with the quantitative limits and the qualitative inadequacy of the necessary [physical] means, so that their satisfaction requires planful provision and work, struggle with nature and the association of human beings" (1949, 63–64).

## The Protestant Ethic and the Spirit of Capitalism

One of the questions that Weber asks himself is, not unexpectedly, similar to one of the questions Marx asks himself: What explains the beginning of capitalism in Western European economic organizations? What broke the centuries-long tradition of feudalism in that part of the world?[19] More generally, "how [can] anything new . . . ever arise in this world [which is] oriented . . . toward the *regular* as the empirically valid?" Weber's answer to both questions is the same: It is *charisma*—the charisma of human individuals—that explains *the end (termination) of feudalism*. But because charisma is itself "naturally unstable" (1978, 1114) and because it naturally destabilizes all established ways, and also because it soon destabilizes its own destabilization, "when the tide that lifted a charismatically led group out of everyday life flows back into the channels of workaday routines, at least the 'pure' form of charismatic domination will wane and turn into an 'institution'" (1978, 1121). Because the participants in a charismatic movement are living biological organisms requiring regular and frequent subsistence from outside themselves, "the most fundamental problem is that of making a transition from a charismatic administrative staff, and the corresponding principles of administration, to one which is adapted to everyday conditions. . . . [rather than living on irregular] gifts, booty, or sporadic acquisition" (1978, 253, 249).

For this reason, "charismatic authority . . . *cannot remain stable*, but becomes *either traditionalized or rationalized*, or a combination of both" (1978, 246; see also 249, 250, 251; 1951b, 113; cf. Schluchter 1989, 403). This turning point between the destabilizing shock of charisma, on the one hand, and the restabilizing processes of traditionalization and rationalization, on the other hand, takes on acute sociocultural consequences "with the disappearance of the personal charismatic leader and with the [emergence of the] problem of *succession*" (1978, 246)—involving at least the participant-outlet institution. Here Weber sees several "principal types of solution," including "the concept that charisma may . . . become the *charisma of office*" (1978, 248)—an office that almost noncharismatic individuals may fill.

## Propulsion, and Steering, at the Point of Charismatic Destabilization

Now consider the more general question—namely, what explains whether a culture structure, once *destabilized* by the random shock of charisma, turns to a *new* stable stage or turns back to an *old* stable stage?

Weber answers: "not *ideas*, but material and *ideal interests, directly govern man's conduct* [he does not tell us the difference between an idea and an interest]. Yet very frequently the 'world images' that have been created by 'ideas' have, like switchmen, determined the *tracks* along which action has been pushed by the dynamic of interest" (1946, 280).

In addition, says Weber, there is human psychical inertia: "A man does not 'by nature' wish to earn more and more money, but simply to live as he is accustomed to live and to earn as much as is necessary for that purpose.[20] Wherever modern capitalism has begun . . . it has encountered the immensely stubborn resistance of this leading trait of pre-capitalistic labor." This inertia, Weber claims, caused both carrot and stick to fail: "the appeal to higher wage-rates failed [as did forcing] the worker by reduction of his wage-rates to work harder to earn the same amount [as] he did before" (1958, 60).

Something (in addition to the constant competitiveness quoted above in note 20) there was powerful enough, however, to overcome this inertia and to produce capitalism—and this "something" was the individual's religious fear of God: specifically, self-interest in the possibility of one's own supernatural salvation and eternal life: "The only way of living acceptably to God," and thereby achieving that personal salvation and everlasting life, was "solely through the *fulfillment of the obligations [to God] imposed upon the individual by his position in the world. That [obligation] was his calling*" (1958, 80).

To Martin Luther's (1483-1546) charismatic idea of an individual's *"calling"* or divinely determined vocation, Weber says, John Calvin (1509-1564) added "the doctrine of [an individual's] *predestination*"—namely, that "by the decree of [the omniscient and omnipotent] God . . . some men and angels are predestined unto everlasting life, and others foreordained to everlasting death" (1958, 100), and there is simply no effect that any human actions can have on that destiny. "God's grace is . . . as impossible for those to whom He has granted it to lose as it is unattainable for those to whom He has denied it" (1958, 104).

Therefore, Weber concludes, "The question 'Am I one of the elect?' must sooner or later have arisen for every believer and have forced all other interests into the background. And how can I be sure of this state of grace?" (1958, 110)—this was the self-*interest rationality* (*Zweckrationalität*) question of personal immortality.

Enter the pastors of Lutheran congregations as rational routinizers (though perhaps not self-consciously so) of Luther's and Calvin's charisma.[21] Pastors

> met [the] difficulties [of self-interest uncertainty—i.e., the question "Am I one of the elect?"] in various ways. So far as predestination was not reinterpreted, toned down, or fundamentally abandoned. . . . On the one hand it is held to be an absolute duty to *consider oneself chosen*, and to combat all doubts as temptations of the devil, since lack of self-confidence is the result of insufficient faith, hence of imperfect grace. . . . On the other hand, in order *to attain that self-confidence worldly activity is recommended as the most suitable means*. It and it alone disperses religious doubts and gives the certainty of grace. (1958, 111–112)

But we have seen Marx argue that capitalist "worldly activity" comes in two antithetical sociocultural roles, one of which is employing, and the other is being available for employment—and Weber sees this difference as a matter of psychical behavior tendencies that are then reflected in physical behaviors. For the directing employers, Weber says, "everything is done in terms of balances: at the beginning of the enterprise an initial balance, before every individual decision a *calculation* to ascertain its probably profitableness, and at the end a final balance to ascertain how much profit has been made" (1958, 18). For the implementing employees, however, "in general . . . an attitude which, at least during working hours, is *freed from continual calculations* of how the customary wage may be earned with a maximum of comfort and a minimum of exertion" (1958, 62) is appropriate. In short, the Protestant ethic sponsored a distinctive culture structural "spirit" (that is, a combined "calling" and "predestination") for each of the two Marxian classes in capitalist economic organizations.

But how could a person find out to which of these classes he/she belongs? The answer, Weber says, lies in the person's paying strict attention to his/her God-given worldly *opportunity*: "If God show you a way in which you may lawfully get more than in any other way (without wrong to your soul or to any other), if you refuse this, and choose the less gainful way, you cross one of the ends of your calling, and you refuse to be God's steward." If you *see no such opportunity*, then *"faithful labor*, even at low wages, on the part of those whom life offers no other opportunities, is highly pleasing to God" (1958, 162, 178).

It should be no surprise, then, that Weber tells us that "with great regularity we find the most genuine adherents of Puritanism among the classes which were *rising* from a lowly status" (1958, 174) because individuals belonging to a rising group would be more likely to see opportunities to "get more" than were members of falling groups.

The net result of Weber's argument in *The Protestant Ethic and the Spirit of Capitalism*, then, is that *not a Marxian role-conflict but a Durkheimian role-complementarity* evolved in the minds of both employers and employees—such that *employees'* "*work was becoming a [religiously sanctified] calling*" and also "*employer's acquisition of money [from employees' work, was becoming] another [such] 'calling'*" (2002, 121). Not Marxian secular class conflict but Weberian sacred class cooperation (and a Durkheimian cross between the two) became the Protestant order of the day.

Put in more specifically Weberian terms, the capitalistic economic division of labor was made sacred by a burst of charismatic attribution toward the preachings of Martin Luther and John Calvin, and these individuals' leadership of their religious organizations conferred divine honor and self-confidence on *both* classes of congregants. In other words, to the "indispensable ethical qualities of the modern capitalist *entrepreneur* . . . [were added the equally indispensable ethical qualities of the] *worker's* special will for work" (1951, 247).

Finally, one notes that the power of the religious organizations set forth by Weber inheres in congregants' church-supported role-differences in this-world and also in the afterworld: "Strata with high social and economic privilege . . . assign to religion the primary function of legitimizing their own life pattern and situation in the world. . . . Correspondingly different is the situation of the disprivileged. Their particular need is for release from suffering. . . . [The] hope for and expectation of just compensation, a fairly calculating attitude, is, next to magic (indeed, not unconnected with it), the most widely diffused form of mass religion all over the world" (1978, 491–492, italics removed).

## *The Routinization of Charisma: Bureaucracy and Machinery*

The routinization period that follows the sudden deroutinizing shock of charisma is accomplished, Weber says, by nonrational "traditionalization or [rational] legalization. . . . In the first case a prebendal organization [where subsistence allowances are made to members by the state] will result; in the second, patrimonialism or bureaucracy" (1978, 250). In Weber's view, the latter outcome is so superior in its other-interest rationality (*Wertrationalität*) that he tells us "*the future belongs to bureaucratization*" (1978, 1401; see also Beetham 1985, 71)—as Marx believes the future belongs to robotic mechanization. To Weber, "where administration has been completely bureaucratized, the resulting system of domination is practically indestructible. The individual bureaucrat cannot squirm out of the apparatus into which he has been harnessed. . . . [and the] ruled . . . cannot dispense with or replace the bureaucratic apparatus once it exists" (1978, 987–988).

To this, Weber adds, by way of characterizing both machines and bureaucracies, that "the primary source of the superiority of bureaucratic administration lies in the role of [the scientific education organizational] *technical knowledge* which, through the development of modern [machine] technology and [bureaucratic] business methods in the production of goods, has become completely indispensable. . . . Bureaucratic administration means fundamentally domination through [scientific] knowledge" (1978, 223, 225; see also 1417–1418)—as does mechanization. Thus, Weber tells us that "*Together with the non-living machine . . . that animated machine, the bureaucratic organization, with its specialization of trained skills, its division of jurisdiction, its rules and hierarchical relations of authority . . . is busy fabricating the shell of bondage which men will perhaps be forced to inhabit some day as powerless as the fellahs of ancient Egypt*" (1978, 1402).

Weber seems to have forgotten, however, in these last forecasts, his own claims that "in a revolutionary and sovereign manner, *charismatic domination* transforms *all* values and breaks *all* traditional and rational norms" and, by implication, then, *all* "shells of bondage"—including its own. He is forgetting his forecast that charisma "threatens to happen *everywhere*," and he is forgetting that all these statements imply *permanently recurring change* in human sociocultural phenomena.[22]

In this way, Weber leaves us with two opposing, long-term forecasts regarding the survival of the human species—one forecast of endless "bondage" to bureaucracy and inanimate machinery, and one of endlessly recurrent charismatic bondage breaking.

## Chapter 5

## THE SUPPLEMENTAL THEORIES OF IBN KHALDÛN AND OTHERS: GEOGRAPHY AND TECHNOLOGY

Chapters 3 and 4 examined Marx's and Weber's supplements to Durkheim's core sociological theory (chapter 2)—supplements which they make by focusing on *the human individual participants'* physical and psychical behavior capacities, respectively, as nonsociocultural (i.e., species biological) constituent influences *inside* human sociocultural phenomena. The present chapter shifts the focus to Ibn Khaldûn's (and others') emphasis on two *outside, environmental* influences on those phenomena.

The environments in question are, first, the "natural" *geographical* (and, more inclusively, solar systemic and cosmic) phenomena from which empirical science says single-celled Earthly life—and eventually our own complex life—evolved, and from which all life daily draws its entire subsistence. The second outside environment comprises "artificial," human-made *technological* constructions with which humans have modified their geographical environments and themselves.[1]

There are at least two basic reasons why we have to take these environmental factors into account in a book about classical sociological thoughts pertaining to human species survival. The first reason is that physical thermodynamics tells us no macrolevel phenomenon, whether sociocultural or nonsociocultural, can continue to manifest a given causal effect without periodically *replacing* the energy expended in that manifestation from some other, environing, source—otherwise the causal factor (including, ultimately, the universe as a whole) simply runs down and becomes incapable of continuing to produce that effect. This is why chapter 1 defined societies as participant-*throughput* systems, and therefore as *self-replenishing* systems. It is why Marx makes the economic (subsistence-producing) labor-power and instruments of production the centerpieces of his theory. It is why Durkheim himself says "all forces . . . are worn away with the passage of time if nothing replenishes the energy they lose in the ordinary course of events"—thereby (but perhaps unconsciously) opening his own sociocultural *self-maintenance* thesis to the necessity of energy-*replenishment from outside.*

Second, with the now experimentally confirmed exception of quantum entanglement (see Gribbin 1995, 223; Greene 2004, 105–123), all the phenomena that the empirical sciences have so far identified as causes of other phenomena produce their effects only through some *transmitting* phenomenon that "carries" the causal energy outward from those causes, ultimately, to the rest of the universe at large.

We begin this chapter by examining Ibn Khaldûn's reliance on the same social structural and culture structural mechanisms as Durkheim, Marx, and Weber do, to assure ourselves that he is talking about the same kinds of phenomena we are.

## *Social Structure and Culture Structure*

Abdurahman Muhammad Ibn Khaldûn[2] tells us that "man is distinguished from the other living beings by . . . [the] ability to *think* . . . [and by] Man's efforts to *make a living*" (1969, 42)—thereby implying the coexistence of culture structure and social structure. Then, identifying "the power of thinking" with "'*rational* power,'" Ibn Khaldûn implies a definition of "rationality" that accords with what Weber calls "objective" (empirical scientific) rationality insofar as it relies on "the powers of external sense perception, with the organs of vision, hearing, and all the other (organs), [leading] up to inward (perception)" and then "the estimative [that is, forecasting] power and the power of memory" (1969, 76; see also 83–89 regarding *dreaming* as a further type of thought). Ibn Khaldûn, however, does not mention the "*inter*subjectivity," the group consensuality, that Weber regards as indispensable to empirical scientific ("objective") rationality.

Ibn Khaldûn also refers to the culture structural factor of "prestige" (Weber's term is "charisma") as "an *accident* that affects human beings [and that] comes into being and decays inevitably," but Ibn Khaldûn implies accidents can be socioculturally routinized when he tells us that *systematically inherited* "royal authority [is] the greatest possible kind of glory and prestige" (1969, 105, 112).

Then, exemplifying human "powers of [physical] *action*" and therefore, implicitly, social structure, Ibn Khaldûn cites "touching with the hand, walking with the foot, speaking with the tongue, and the total combined motion with the body" (1969, 76)—anticipating Weber's abbreviation "my hand tips my hat."

### Culture Structural Group Feeling

A central concept in Ibn Khaldûn's theory is "group feeling," a morality *culture structure* that anticipates Durkheim's "social solidarity," Marx's "class consciousness," and Weber's "Protestant ethic" and "spirit of capitalism"—except that Ibn Khaldûn bases "group feeling" on *kinship* relationships—which none of the others do. "(Respect for) *blood ties*," Ibn Khaldûn says, "is something natural among men, with the rarest exceptions. It leads to affection for one's relations and blood relatives, (the feeling that) no harm ought to befall them nor any destruction come upon them. One feels shame when one's relatives are treated unjustly or attacked, and one wishes to intervene between them and whatever peril or destruction threatens them."

Ibn Khaldûn, however, immediately relaxes this "natural" kinship restriction: "*Clients and allies* belong in the same category [as blood relatives]. The affection everybody has for his clients and allies results from the feeling of shame that comes to a person when one of his neighbors, relatives, or a blood relation in any degree is humiliated" (1969, 98). So, in Ibn Khaldûn's view, what holds kinship groups, clients and patrons, allies, and neighbors together in a society is culture structural "prestige," "group feeling," shared "charisma" attribution from each member to every other member—in a particular geographical and technological habitat (as we shall see in a moment).

To this, Ibn Khaldûn adds that "*group feeling . . . depends on numerical strength . . .* [and the] real reason why (large dynasties last longer than smaller ones) is that when collapse comes it begins in the [geographically] outlying regions . . . the large dynasty has many such provinces far from its centre" (1969, 130), and that "a dynasty is stronger at its centre than at its border regions" (1969, 128; cf. Wallerstein 1979).

## *Social Structural Force and Violence*

Then, to culture structural "*group feeling,*" and social structural "*numerical strength,*" Ibn Khaldûn adds social structural *physical force and violence* (already implicit in "numerical strength"). Thus,

> people find it difficult to submit to general dynastic (power) at the beginning, unless they are *forced* into

submission by [their enemies'] strong superiority. . . . But once leadership is firmly vested in the members of the family qualified to exercise royal authority in the dynasty, and once (royal authority) has been passed on by inheritance over many generations and through successive dynasties, the beginnings are forgotten, and the members of that family are clearly marked [culture structurally] as leaders. It has become a firmly established article of [culture structural] faith that one must be [social structurally] subservient and submissive to them.... It is as if obedience to the government were a divinely revealed book that cannot be changed or opposed. (1969, 123–124)

## *The Rise and Fall of Ruling "Houses" and Dynasties*

Ibn Khaldûn claims social structural cooperation is *required* for the survival of Homo sapiens: "It is *absolutely necessary* for [an individual] man to have the cooperation of his fellow-men" both for obtaining "food or nourishment" and for self-defense. Without cooperation, Ibn Khaldûn says, "the human species would vanish" (1969, 46). But cooperation is always met by resistance: "*aggressiveness* is natural in living beings" (1969, 46), and here again, superior cooperative force inhibits other force: "Mutual aggression of people in towns and cities [against each other] is averted by the authorities and the government, which hold back the masses under their control from attacks and aggression upon each other. They are thus prevented by the influence of force and governmental authority from mutual injustice, save such injustice as comes from the ruler himself" (1969, 97–98).

Because of the (social structural) power and (culture structural) prestige of such authority, there is "great competition for [royal authority]. It rarely is handed over (voluntarily), but it may be taken away [by force]. Thus, discord ensues. It leads to war and fighting, and to attempts to gain superiority" (1969, 123). However, when royal authority is peacefully inherited under sociocultural constraints, the inheritors are called first a "house," then, after many generations, [the "house"] is called a "dynasty": "A 'house' means that a man counts noble and famous [Weber would say charismatic] men among his forebears. The fact that he is their progeny and descendant gives him great standing among his fellows" (1969, 102)—and so "a 'house' possesses an original nobility through group feeling and personal qualities"—but "later on, the people (who have a 'house') divest themselves of that nobility when group feeling disappears as the result of sedentary life, and they mingle with the common people" (1969, 102).

## Alternation of Appetite and Forgetfulness, and the Use of Physical Force

Indeed, Ibn Khaldûn claims that rise-and-fall is a general regularity of existence: "The [geographical] world of the elements and all it contains comes into being and decays. Minerals, plants, all the animals including man, and the other created things come into being and decay. . . . Sciences grow up and then are wiped out. The same applies to [technology-inventing] crafts, and to similar things" (1969, 105). "Time," he says, "gets the upper hand over the original group (in power [within a society]). Their prowess disappears as a result of senility. . . . They reach their limit, the limit that is set by the nature of human urbanization and political superiority. . . . Royal authority thus continues in a particular nation until the force of its group feeling is broken and gone, or until all its groups have ceased to exist" (1969, 114–115).

Behind this rise-and-fall pattern of human sociocultural phenomena, Ibn Khaldûn says, there lies a similar pattern of culture structure—specifically, a shared feeling of *appetite* which build up, followed by a *forgetfulness* of the effort that it took to build up (compare Pareto's similarly culture structural cyclical alternation, in the political organizations of a society, of "the lions and the foxes" [1935, paragraphs 2178–2179]).

Thus, appetite drives the pursuit of bare necessities of subsistence up through the nomadic way of life to the pursuit of luxuries through the sedentary way of life. Then slowly forgetfulness begins to take over:

> The builder of the family's glory knows what it cost him to do the work, and he keeps the qualities that created his glory and made it last. The son who comes after him had personal contact with his father and thus learned those things from him. . . . The third generation must be content with imitation and, in particular, with reliance upon tradition. . . . The fourth generation . . . imagines that the edifice was not built through application and effort. . . . For [a member of that generation] sees the great respect in which he is held by the people, but he does not know how that respect originated and what the reason for it was. He imagines that it is due to his descent and nothing else. (1969, 105–106)

In sum: "The four generations can be defined as the builder, the one who has personal contact with the builder, the one who relies on tradition, and the destroyer" (1969, 106)—whereupon a new four-generation dynastic cycle (one builder generation; two maintainer generations; one destroyer generation) may begin, end, and be succeeded by another such cycle involving different participants, owing to participant-throughput.

*War*, a violently forceful relationship between societies, originates in an appetitive—imperialistic—culture: "the origin of war," Ibn Khaldûn says, is "as a rule either jealousy and envy, or hostility, or zeal in behalf of God and His religion, or zeal in behalf of royal authority and the effort to found a kingdom" (1958, 73; see also 298). That "effort to found a kingdom" is forcefully expansionist—that is, it employs "dynastic war against seceders and those who refuse obedience," and Ibn Khaldûn refers to "wars against Arab and Berber nations, in order to force them into submission" (1958, 74) and to build from those submissions an empire.[3]

One realizes that Ibn Khaldûn is proposing a human species survival mechanism based on geography and military technology that is different from those we have seen in Malthus, Darwin, Durkheim, Marx, and Weber. That mechanism is *military conquest*—that is, one population's forceful and violent effort to incorporate another population's habitat into its own (a proposition that Spencer later adopted for his theory—see chapter 2, note 4).

## *Geography and Technology in Human Sociocultural Life*

Ibn Khaldûn's special early contribution to classical sociological theory is the hypothesis that nonhuman and nonsociocultural *geography* (natural habitat) and *technology* (constructed, or artificial, habitat) are major influences on all human sociocultural phenomena. Thus, Ibn Khaldûn tells us that "the earth has a spherical shape and is enveloped by the element of water. It may be compared to a grape floating upon water. . . . The part of the earth that is free from water and thus suitable for human civilization has more waste and empty areas than (habitable) areas. The empty area in the south is larger than in the north. The [socioculturally] cultivated part of the earth extends more toward the north" (1969, 49). There is, Ibn Khaldûn says, "little civilization [near the equator]. There is a medium degree of civilization [somewhat north of the equator] because the heat there is temperate owing to the decreased amount of light. There is a great deal of civilization [still farther north of the equator] because of the decreased amount of heat there," but in the extreme north "generation stops because of the excessive cold and frost and the long time without any heat" (1967, 107, 106).

Moderate climatic heat, then, is a strong explanatory variable in Ibn Khaldûn's theory because, he says, "excessive heat causes a parching dryness in the air that prevents [biological] generation. As the heat becomes more excessive, water and all kinds of moisture dry up. . . . [After that,] the heat becomes more or less temperate. Then, generation can take place. This goes on until the cold becomes excessive, due to the lack of light and the obtuse angles of the rays of the sun. Then generation again decreases and is destroyed" (1969, 56). In short, Ibn Khaldûn pre-echoes Ward and Brownlee's later and much larger-scaled "Location! Location! Location! [That is the] secret for . . . populating the Universe. Much of the Universe is clearly hostile to life, and only rare places offer even potential oases for its existence" (2000, 15).

Ibn Khaldûn concludes that "the different [sociocultural] ways in which [people] make their living" (1969, 91)—and the extents to which they are successful in doing so—depend not on genotypic differences between the people but on differences between the peoples' geographical habitats and their technologies. These are, in turn, consequences of what the present author has called the "luck of the territorial draw" (see Wallace 1997, 15–19) as groups of Homo sapiens migrated out of East Africa perhaps 200,000 years ago, and settled at various distances from their common starting point perhaps because otherwise hospitable intervening locations had already been settled.

Ibn Khaldûn, knowing nothing of these prehistoric migrations of our species, of course, refers to its later settlements: "[Peoples] who live by agriculture or animal husbandry cannot avoid the call of the desert, because it alone offers wide fields, pastures for animals, and other things that the settled areas do not offer. . . . Subsequent improvement of their conditions and acquisition of more wealth and comfort than they need, cause them to rest and take it easy. . . . They build [technologically] large houses, and lay out towns and cities for protection. . . . Sedentary people means the inhabitants of cities and countries, some of whom adopt the [technology-creating] crafts as their way of making a living, while others adopt commerce" (1969, 91–92).[4]

There are, in short, Ibn Khaldûn says, "*desert* (Bedouin) civilization as found in outlying regions and mountains, in hamlets near pastures in waste regions, and on the fringes of sandy deserts; [and] . . . *sedentary* civilization as found in cities, villages, towns, and small communities that serve the purpose of protection and fortification by means of walls" (1969, 43).[5]

Regarding the technological idea that "cities, villages, towns, and small communities . . . serve the purpose of *protection and fortification by means of walls*" (1969, 43), Ibn Khaldûn argues, again, in favor of cyclical rise-and-fall development: "When cities are first founded, they have few dwellings and few building materials. . . . Then the [sociocultural] civilization of a city grows and its inhabitants increase in number. Now the [technological] materials used for (building) increase, because of the increase in (available) labor and the increased number of craftsmen. (This process goes on) until (the city) reaches the limit in that respect. The civilization of the city then recedes, and its inhabitants decrease in number" (1969, 272).[6] After every rise there comes a fall; human history (even cosmic history) has its ups and downs.

Let us turn now to some of the more recent inheritors of Ibn Khaldûn's concern with the impact of geographical and technological factors on human sociocultural phenomena.

## Some Theoretical Descendants of Ibn Khaldûn's View of Geography

Although geographical and technological factors are far from the centerpieces of Weber's theory, he calls on both these factors repeatedly for explanation of human sociocultural phenomena. For example, "in the [German] west and south bottoms, river valleys, and plateaux, are intermingled" so the people there produce and exchange different goods, while "in the east . . . the neighboring towns have much more frequently nothing to exchange with each other . . . [because they have] the same geographical situation [and] produce the same goods" (1958b, 366, 377–378).[7]

More recently, Lenski argues that not only has geography facilitated certain sociocultural developments, but "the ecology of a particular area has prevented [the inhabitants] from adopting new technologies: much of sub-Saharan Africa, for example, seems to have been unsuited to the plow under preindustrial conditions.—The combination of poor soil and the presence of the tsetse fly (which severely limited the areas in which cattle and horses could be raised) virtually ruled out the use of the plow before the development of modern commercial fertilizers and chemical insecticides. . . . The geographical distribution of simple societies in the modern world, with their concentration in deserts, rain forests, and arctic areas, is no mere accident of history, nor does it reflect some curious distribution of values" (1975, 147). Similarly, Zinsser points out that the temporal and spatial distributions of natural predators on human life have had profound sociocultural impacts:

> Civilizations have retreated from the plasmodium of malaria, and armies have crumpled into rabbles under the onslaught of cholera spirilla, or of dysentery and typhoid bacilli. Huge areas have been devastated by the trypanosome that travels on the wings of the tsetse fly, and generations have been harassed by the syphilis of a courtier. . . . [Rats] destroy cultivated grains . . . destroy merchandise . . . poultry [and] enormous numbers of eggs. . . . [They] have gnawed holes in dams and started floods; they have started fires by gnawing matches; they have bitten holes in mail sacks and eaten the mail; they have actually caused famines in India by wholesale crop destruction in scant years. (1967, 6, 151)

Diamond asks, "Why was the ancient rate of technological and political development fastest in Eurasia, slower in the Americas (and in Africa south of the Sahara), and slowest in Australia?" and he answers that the differences stemmed "ultimately from continental differences in geography" (1999, 235, 237; see also Sowell 1996, 9–19). Diamond then adds that "the striking differences between the long-term histories of peoples of the different continents have been due not to innate differences in the peoples themselves but to differences in their [geographical] environments. . . . [T]he same ancestral peoples either ended up extinct, or returned to living as hunter-gatherers, or went on to build complex states, depending on their [geographical] environments" (1999, 405–406; see also Sowell 1996, 9–19).

And still more recently, Fagan tells us, "Today, we are experiencing sustained [global] warming of a kind unknown since the Ice Age. And this warming is certain to bring drought—sustained drought and water shortages" (2008, 239). Drought, Fagan says, "is the silent and insidious killer associated with global warming. . . . [B]y 2010 around 300 million people in sub-Saharan Africa . . . will suffer from malnutrition because of intensifying drought. . . . By 2025, an estimated 2.8 *billion* of us will live in areas with increasingly scarce water resources" (2008, 233, italics in original). Fagan continues: "Drought and water are probably the overwhelmingly important issue for this and future centuries, times when we will have to become accustomed to making altruistic decisions that will benefit not necessarily ourselves but generations yet unborn. . . . And a great deal of long-term thinking will have to involve massive investments [from the more developed world to] the developing world, for it is most at risk" (2008, 240–241).

## Some Theoretical Descendants of Ibn Khaldûn's View of Technology

Of technology, Weber says: "A certain degree of development of the means of communication ... is one of the most important prerequisites for the possibility of bureaucratic administration"; and "war in our time," he says, "is a war of machines, and this makes central provisioning necessary, just as the dominance of the machine in industry promotes the concentration of the means of production and management"; "By contrast [with the Orient], all . . . city unions of the Occident . . . were coalitions of armed strata of the cities. This was the decisive difference" (1978, 973, 981, 1262).

Durkheim, too, has something to say for technological factors (but not much for geographical factors) as influences on sociocultural phenomena: "material things . . . play an essential role in the common life. . . . [For example,] avenues of communication which have been constructed before our time give a definite direction to our lives, depending on whether they connect us with one or another country" (1951, 314), and we have already seen his claim that technology offers significantly more opportunities to commit suicides "by throwing one's self from a high place . . . in great cities than in the country: the *buildings* are higher."

Chapter 3 pointed out the heavy causal weight Marx assigns to technology. He argues that "slavery cannot be abolished without the steam-engine and the mule and spinning jenny, serfdom cannot be abolished without improved agriculture, and . . . in general, people cannot be liberated as long as they are unable to obtain food and drink, housing and clothing in adequate quality and quantity" (1969, 1:26–27; see also 37). Engels adds that "only at a certain level of development of the productive forces of society . . . does it become possible to raise production to such an extent that the abolition of class distinctions . . . can be lasting without bringing about stagnation and even decline in the mode of social production" (1969, 3:387).

Ogburn argues that "material culture," which is his term for what we are here calling technology—but he includes the human social structural and culture structural design, operation, and maintenance as well as the nonliving instrument itself—and says it affects "changes in other parts of culture such as social organization and customs," and that "the introduction of steam makes changes in home production, the growth of cities, changes in the position of women, new causes of war" (1933, 196, 270). Cottrell adds that technology determines the amount and kinds of energy available to humans and "the energy available to man limits what he can do and influences what he will do" (1955, 2), while Levy takes "the ratio of non-living to animate sources of power" as "the [single best] measure of modernization" (1972, 3), and White tells us that "the primary role [in human society] is played by the technological system . . . culture as a whole is dependent upon the [technological] material, mechanical means of adjustment to the [geographical] natural environment" (1949, 364, 365).

Ong points out that literacy is "a *technology . . . a matter of tools outside us*" (1971, 6), and that the effects of these tools on cultural structure are different from those of the spoken word (that is, orality—which we, but apparently not Ong, regard as also a technology, a matter of tools, specifically sound waves, outside us): "Writing is an absolute necessity for the analytically sequential, linear organization of thought. . . . Without writing . . . the mind simply cannot engage in this sort of thinking, which is unknown in primary oral cultures, where thought is exquisitely elaborated, not in analytic linearity, but in formulary fashion, through 'rhapsodizing,' that is, stitching together proverbs, antitheses, epithets, and other 'commonplaces'" (1971, 2). In addition, Ong claims that "an oral culture must maintain its knowledge by repeating it," and consequently "originality threatens [such a culture with] disaster as it no longer need do when writing can store or 'park' knowledge outside the mind for any future use as needed, freeing noetic powers for pursuit of new thoughts" (1971, 3).

In similar manner, Goody and Watt argue that in literate societies, people "are faced with permanently recorded versions of the past and its beliefs; and because the past is thus set apart from the present, historical enquiry becomes possible. This in turn encourages skepticism; and skepticism not only about the legendary past, but about received ideas about the universe as a whole. From here the next step is to see how to build up and test alternative explanations" (1972, 353)—and of course we would add to test, with the technology of computer simulations, alternative *forecasts* of events and alternative *preparations* for those events.

Gouldner says that "the culture of discourse that produces ideology was historically grounded in the technology of a specific kind of mass (or public) media, [namely,] printing," but when one watches television, "one is not commonly left with a sense that one needs to do something actively after a viewing. The viewing is an end in itself" (1976, 39, 168)—although Gouldner offers neither evidence nor hypothetical explanation for this presumed difference. And Erikson notes that "today . . . we no longer parade deviants in the town square . . . but it is interesting that the 'reform' which brought about this change in penal practice coincided almost exactly with the development of *newspapers* as a medium of mass information. . . . Newspapers (and now radio and television) offer much the same kind of entertainment as public hangings or a Sunday visit to the local gaol" (1966, 12).

Jastrow speculates that an evolutionary step toward a species successor to Homo sapiens may become possible through advances in what Marx calls the "instruments of labor": "a new form of life is being created today in the laboratory of the computer scientist. It is an artificial life, made out of silicon chips rather than neurons. . . . We will see the silicon brain as an emergent form of life, competitive with man" (1981, 91, 144). A couple of years earlier, Hogan argued that

> a man is aware of himself as existing in the localized region of space that is defined as the focal point of his senses. [A conceivable artificial intelligence, however,]

will perceive the universe through billions of sensory channels distributed all over the surface of the Earth and beyond. On top of that, its "senses" [could] cover the whole spectrum from high-power proton microscopes in research labs to the big orbiting astronomic telescopes . . . from galactic gravity-wave detectors to the infrared sensors lowered into the ocean trenches. . . . [Such] an intelligence, controlling robot extensions, [could move] pieces of itself around in millions of places at one time [on Jupiter,] under the Arctic ice caps. . . . How can we even begin to imagine how an awareness as totally alien as that would perceive itself and the universe around it? (1979, 65)

## *Military and Police Political Technology*

Across the roughly five thousand years of human civilization so far, it has become virtually impossible to overlook the sociocultural roles of the specialized technology of intersocietal *warfare and weapons*, but except for Spencer's and Weber's (see 1978, 1150–1155), there are not many references to warfare or to weapons in the works of classical sociological theorists. Ferguson, however, tells us that "we are now [only in] the second decade of *archaeology's* discovery of war" (2006, 469)—thereby indicating that sociology has not been alone in paying little attention to war and weapons. Based on evidence of "archaeology's [recent] discovery of war," however, Ferguson concludes that "war seems absent in the Paleolithic, and emerges first with more settled [Neolithic] foragers (although most of them were peaceable)" (2006, 469, 473).

Ferguson rejects the idea that "war is something . . . that all humans [instinctively] do" and proposes, instead, six "preconditions" (all but the last are sociocultural, though not so named) that made "the origin and/or the intensification of war more likely." These preconditions are: "a shift to sedentary existence," "increasing population within broad areas," "the development of social ranking," "increasing trade, especially of status goods," "the development of social institutions for bounding groups in conflict," and "a serious ecological reversal, involving climate change or anthropogenic resource degradation"—to which Ferguson adds that "over the millennia, these preconditions became more widespread, and war arose in more regions of the world" (2006, 496, 497).

Speaking of the early river-valley civilizations of the late Neolithic—those of Mesopotamia, Egypt, the Indus, the Yangtze, and Peru, Ferguson tells us that "Relatively stable, central states, the sources of our earliest histories, commonly saw themselves as surrounded by fierce 'barbarians' . . . [and] militaristic states, over time, replaced comparatively non-militaristic ones" (2006, 498). "Then came the European expansion. . . . Europeans crossed enormous distances and oceans. Doing this, they introduced new diseases, plants, and animals that massively disrupted contacted groups. Europeans had trade goods that were in great demand . . . and military and transportation technology and techniques that could revolutionize warfare" (2006, 499).

Specifically regarding the development of weaponry, Brodie and Brodie anticipate Ferguson's remark on the recency of "archaeology's discovery of war" when they say:

> The slowness of weapons progress prior to the nineteenth and especially the twentieth centuries . . . [is explainable, partly, by the fact that] what science there was, and what talent there was for invention, seem often to be dedicated to other pursuits than new weapons, and in fact to have avoided that field. . . . [For two ex-

amples,] Isaac Newton knew nothing of guns, carried out no experiments in gunnery, and had only the slightest interest in the technological application of the great mathematical discoveries [he] recorded . . . [and the father of modern chemistry, Robert Boyle] made clear that he thought no learned man should contribute to the "hellish machines" of destruction and showered bounties upon one scientist who had invented a new explosive to keep him from selling it. (1962, 8, 85, 90)

Fortification seems likely to have been a Neolithic invention—an effective defense by sedentary urban populations against attacks by more mobile parties of attackers: "Nineveh, constructed in 2000 B.C., had stone walls 50 miles long, 120 feet high and 30 feet thick. The Great Wall of China, built in 200 B.C., was twenty feet high and continued for 1,400 miles" (1962, 19–20). And although weapons made especially for attacking such fortifications came into use (e.g., battering rams, movable towers, catapults), "by [A.D.] 1300 defense was so superior to offense that the only certain weapon in siegecraft was famine. Moreover, invading armies, interested chiefly in plunder, could seldom be persuaded to conduct a year-long siege, so great was the doubt of its success" (1962, 31).

The invention of the cannon, however, reversed this superiority. "The first 'cannon' was probably the Arabian madfaa, a deep wooden bowl holding [gunpowder—invented in China] with the cannon ball balanced on the muzzle-top and popped off by the explosion" (1962, 44). Further developments in cannon made them "more effective than the old siege engines, and castles all over Europe fell before their onslaught" (1962, 49).

Meanwhile, Brodie and Brodie note that a revolution in sea power was effected under the leadership of Henry the Navigator, king of Portugal from 1433 to 1460, who "surrounded himself with mathematicians, astronomers, cosmographers, chartmakers, physicians, and instrument-makers. . . . [They] greatly improved the art of map-making, the science of navigation, and the design of ships . . . [and] made voyaging a national passion" (1962, 62–63). As a result, "A single century—1425–1525—saw the maritime exploration of more than half the globe and the three greatest [terrestrial] voyages in human history, those of Vasco da Gama, Columbus, and Magellan" (1962, 63). Soon, fighting ships carried cannon and strategy changed from a close-range opening salvo and ramming followed by boarding and hand-to-hand fighting to standing off and battering each other with artillery: "the warship was no longer a fort with a garrison of soldiers but an arsenal of guns" (1962, 67).

The eighteenth century, Brodie and Brodie claim, "saw the evolution of the steam engine, the development of iron metallurgy, the shift of fuel from wood to coal, the rise of industrial chemistry, the establishment of a machine industry—that is, machines to make machines—and the first stirrings of the science of electricity. Of all these, none had as spectacular consequences as the invention of the steam engine, which resulted, it has been said, in the first major transformation of human life since the Neolithic [invention of] agriculture" (1962, 119).

From this it followed that "the coming of the railroad and the application of steam to the warship were the two most important [military] strategic developments of the nineteenth century" (1962, 148). With the railroad, "large bodies of troops were moved speedily over tremendous distances" (1962, 149), and with the application of steam to warships, an increase in water speed was attained—although "the necessity of keeping the fleet supplied with fuel acted as a tether . . . [which] England finally solved . . . by establishing coaling bases all over the world" (1962, 154).

Then, "with the twentieth century . . . *science* becomes . . . intertwined with the technology of war" (1962, 172) and quickly produces a string of big inventions in warfare including the airplane, radar, the machine gun, the proximity fuse, the tank, poison gas, the submarine, the ballistic missile, and nuclear weapons (see 1962, 173; see also 200–278). Robotic warfare—in combination with all these innovations—seems still mainly in the planning stage but will, if and when it matures, doubtless be one of the most dangerous of all human-made threats to human sociocultural and species survival.

## *Our Own Long-Term Human Species Survival Forecast*

Finally, we should at least mention the possible utility of technological defenses of human sociocultural phenomena and the human species against truly long-term but cosmically powerful events. In this regard, astrophysicists tell us that in 5–6 billion years our Sun will expand to a size that will swallow, and totally incinerate, the Earth—but long before that, a mere 900 million years from now, the Sun will already have become too hot to allow Earth to continue harboring any currently known form of life at all.

Perhaps on the basis of that forecast but long before that time, the human species will have prepared an astronomical implementation of Darwin's migration-speciation mechanism. Twelve stars are currently listed within a radius of ten to twenty light years of Earth that "could host at least one rocky inner planet suitable for habitation by Earth-type plant and animal life without special environmental protection" (www.solstation.com/stars.htm, "Notable nearby stars"; see also Angier 2008). A series of such planets and their suns—if they are young enough but not too young—might conceivably provide a chain of successive habitats for our species, allowing us to outlast our own homeland and its progenitor Sun.

It is conceivable, then, that as our universe accelerates its expansion, our very distant descendants (of whatever species) may planet-hop until there are simply no more hospitable planets left within their reach. But by then those descendants may be able to construct new life-hospitable planets from materials found in life-inhospitable planets, place the newly constructed planets in appropriate orbits around hospitable stars and migrate to them—until, finally, there are no more such stars.

Perhaps then, the astrophysics that we now know will close our show. Ibn Khaldûn will have been right about rises inexorably foretelling falls, and dust will be not only terrestrial life's first state but its last state too.

# Part III

# Chapter 6

# SUMMARY AND CONCLUSION

Chapter 1 opened with the claim that everything now known to empirical science as lasting any time at all is at least partly *self-maintaining*. For example, every living organism regardless of its species maintains itself by exchanging resources with its geographical environment and through chemical and electrical exchanges among its various organs or organelles. When such exchanges break down for a length of time that exceeds reserves held within the organism, we say the organism dies.

At perhaps the other end of the physical self-maintenance range, a proton (composed of interacting quarks and gluons) is also thought, on theoretical grounds, to eventually terminate its self-maintenance, but experiment has so far only shown that the likely average time of that termination is at least $10^{35}$ years—for all human intents and purposes, permanent.

In any event, Durkheim seems altogether right to nail the "How are sociocultural phenomena self-maintained?" question above the door of the sociology study-room in large letters. And of course we note that this question, not incidentally, welcomes sociobiologists (who study sociocultural phenomena among non-human organisms) as well as sociologists and cultural anthropologists (who study such phenomena among human organisms).

Even though we claim Durkheim was right to apply the hypothesis of *self-maintenance* to human societies, it seems to us wrong to apply *only* that hypothesis to them (it may have seemed wrong to Durkheim too, but that thought may have been suppressed by his vain desire to establish sociology as a science independent of all other sciences—especially psychology). Therefore, we regard Malthus, Darwin, Marx, Weber, and Ibn Khaldûn as going beyond Durkheim's claim that "a social fact cannot be explained except by another *social* fact" to inquire how the innate physical and psychical, proactive as well as reactive, behavior capabilities of *individual members of the human species* contribute to explaining the maintenance of human society, and how the *geographical and technological environments of those individuals* also contribute to that explanation.

## *Proposed Defenses against Species Extinction Threats*

Malthus sees shortages of individual human subsistence as the key threats to human societal and species survival, and he proposes sociocultural *restraint of population size* as the answer to that threat because any *release* of population growth to its natural full potential would lead to subsistence shortages, internecine wars, and to societal extinction and then to species extinction.

We know that Darwin read Malthus's work because he cited it. Darwin's alternative to Malthus's proposed sociocultural population-restraint defense against extinction, however, is to *release* a given population from such restraint while encouraging the resulting excess population to *migrate* out of its homeland to some new geographical location where subsistence is more abundant and competition is less intense. Repeated migrations of this kind would lead to spreading the original species population to new, ever-new, ecological niches around the globe and to adaptive speciations of such life as a whole through its twofold differentiation (that is, differentiations of external habitat and of internal species constitution).

Durkheim poses an alternative to both Malthus's sociocultural population-restraint-*without*-migration-and-*without*-speciation and Darwin's population-release-*with*-migration-and-*with*-speciation extinction defenses. (Durkheim cites Darwin explicitly at 1984, 208–209, but we have not found him citing Malthus anywhere, and the only time we have found him citing Marx is in a book review published after *The Division of Labor*, entitled "Marxism and Sociology: The Materialist Conception of History."[1]) The alternative that Durkheim proposes applies the concept "migration" not to moving surplus human *populations out of existence* (through the restraints that Malthus proposed), or to moving surplus *populations out of competition* (through the geographical and speciation movements that Darwin proposed) to a more abstract sort of migration. Durkheim's migration moves particular human *behaviors out of the repertories of generalist individuals into the repertories of specialist individuals.*

Durkheim argues that his (and Adam Smith's) ideas of labors being distributed among individuals rather than individuals being redistributed among habitats (including existence and nonexistence) can make all participants peaceful cooperators with each other and can permit the entire population to increase in the same habitat by gaining efficiencies of scale in subsistence production and distribution.

There are important differences between the moral culture structures referred to by our theorists, however. Durkheim refers to the evolution of two successive stages of nonconflictful "social solidarity" (first "mechanical" and then "organic") in the participant-organizing organizations of a given society. These stages mandate, in the early stages of human history, relative *unison* in changes from one behavior to another, then in later human history highly differentiated *cooperation* among a society's participants.

Marx, however, claims that both early and late in history, the employers' and employees' "class consciousnesses" mandate social structural *conflict between*, and *cooperation within*, the employer group and their employee groups in economic organizations. This between-group *conflict*, Marx forecasts, diffuses to society's political organizations, which are financially induced to support the employer group against the employee group. When this class-bias becomes intolerable to the employee class, it will forcibly take over the political organizations and after turning that bias around it will introduce the complete automatization of economic production and distribution.

Weber sides with Durkheim's emphasis on sociocultural structures of *cooperation* and *complementarity* between the classes, and against Marx's favoring sociocultural structures of *conflict and dissensus* between them. Thus, Weber argues that these collaborative moralities arose first in the *religious* organizations as one single Protestant "ethic" and then diffused to the economic organizations as two complementary "spirits" of capitalism. Then, rather than leading humankind to the endless future of peace and plenty that Marx foresees, Weber foresees these "spirit[s] of capitalism" leading to an *all-human "bondage"* to culture structures that obey the rules of rationality—apparently forgetting his own prediction that nonrational charisma occurs anywhere and everywhere, and always breaks up fixed regularities—including bondages.

## The Role of Geography and Technology versus Morality Culture Structure

Durkheim credits Adam Smith with being the first to elaborate the theory of the division of labor (of course, Plato was much earlier with *The Republic's* references to a division of labor between "guardians," "warriors," and "commoners"), but we would acknowledge two key elements in Smith's argument that Durkheim passes over without mention—namely, the roles of *geographical* factors and of *technological* factors. On this, Smith tells us, first, that "the improvement in the productive powers of [agricultural] labor . . . does not always keep pace with their improvement in manufactures" because the former is more dependent on the geographically determined *climate* than is the latter. With "the occasions for different sorts of labor [like plowing, harrowing, sowing, and reaping] returning with the *different seasons of the year*," Smith says, "it is impossible that one man should be *constantly* employed in any one of them" (1937, 6). Second, Smith says that although "the division of labor . . . occasions, in every art, a proportionable increase of the productive powers of labor," that increase is brought about by "the necessary *machinery*" (1937, 5; see also 7, 9–10) more than through "improvement of the dexterity of the *workman*" (1937, 7).

In a word, then, Smith argues that if geographical locations, or technological instrumentations, are changed, the human sociocultural division of labor will also change—a point not wasted on Marx, who argues for transforming the *human* division of labor into a human-plus-*machine* division of technology, leaving all living humans free to achieve a finally nonexploitative culture structural diversity undisturbed by species extinction threats.

The special additions to Smith's discussion that Durkheim makes, however, address a different opportunity that the sociocultural division of labor provides—one that rests on Durkheim's claim that the division of labor can be extended beyond the economic organizations to the other participant-organizing organizations of a society—political, religious, and informational—and holds them together, provided that it is supported by a culture structural morality throughout the society that prevents individuals from encroaching on each other's roles and so exploiting them.

Thus, Durkheim tells us that "it is to [the] state of anomie [that is, the absence of an appropriate morality] that . . . must be attributed the continually recurring conflicts and disorder of every kind of which the economic world affords so sorry a spectacle" (cited in chapter 2). So that, to Durkheim, conflict is not a direct consequence of the *presence* of moral directions that tell us to defend contradictory moralities, but it is a default consequence of the *absence* of any moral directions at all—which implies (though he does not say) that humans are innately inclined more toward conflict than toward cooperation.

Indeed, abnormalities in each of Durkheim's two evolutionary stages of cultural morality ("mechanical," and "organic," solidarities) can prey on this innate inclination in two ways. (1) Morality can have a *qualitatively dysfunctional content* (for example, it can direct participants to *harm* rather than help others in the social structure; some of the harmed ones will retaliate; and the conflict that follows will push the society (and the species) a step further toward termination. (2) Morality can be applied with *quantitative immoderation*—that is, its pressure on individual participants can be *too weak* or *too strong*, so that these participants will seek to escape its immoderate pressure through applying suicidal force to themselves, thereby moving their original society and species toward termination. It seems noteworthy that Durkheim does not propose any class biases in suicide rates—although Marx would be the theorist most likely to do so.

## Innate Human Competitiveness and the Class Struggle

Marx argues that the employer–employee division of labor has robbed the vast majority of employees of so much of their life-subsistence as to take away their abilities to adapt to extinction pressures either through Malthusian population-size control or through Darwinian population migration and speciation. They fall victim, then, to a passive, nonresistant, organic solidarity which facilitates their exploitation by employers. The only way out, Marx claims, is leadership of the employee class by an international communist organization which is committed to violent termination of such exploitation.

After that has been accomplished, the combination of *socialism* in the economic organizations and *dictatorship of the proletariat* in the political organizations, Marx says, will permanently wipe out the exploitative employer–employee division of labor from economic, and all other participant-organizing organizations. Next, the new economic and political organizations will together establish a new type of economic division of labor where *all human participants* without regard for previous class status, will be assigned roles formerly reserved for the employer class—namely, *psychical* planning-directing-evaluating work—while allocating to *automatic machines* all the *physical implementation* work formerly assigned to the employee class.

Weber may well have read Marx's forecast of a future division of labor between all human beings as psychical planners-directors-evaluators and automatic machines as physical producers (Weber cites Marx several times—see 1978: 516, 777, 872, 874, 1091), and he says *both* that nonrational charisma can occur *randomly* and when it does occur it is "indeed the specifically *creative* revolutionary force of history," and *also* that bureaucracy will become a "shell of *bondage*" for all humankind (see above).

Weber (and to some extent Ibn Khaldûn), then, halfheartedly warns us against viewing human sociocultural and species life as a foregone certainty. There may be factors in the universe that we have not imagined yet, some of these almost surely occur randomly and may permit our species to survive long after expectations.

Figure 6.1 combines the essential mechanisms for human species survival as implied in Malthus's, Darwin's, Durkheim's, Marx's, Weber's, and Ibn Khaldûn's theories.

One notes, of course, that even when taken all together, the theories examined here are not exhaustive of the presently known dangers to the continued survival of Homo sapiens, and we should expect still more dangers to be discovered and brought under examination in the future. (Ward and Brownlee say that "perhaps we have only begun to see the demons surrounding us as we take our first tentative peeks through our planetary bedroom window into space" [2000:286]—to which we would add that that "space" is both cosmologically outer and socioculturally inner.) For example, none of the classical theories discussed here includes mutually devastating intersocietal or intrasocietal wars, genocides, radical and irreversible global climate changes, uncontrollable disease pandemics, large asteroid strikes, magnetars (see Ward and Brownlee 2000, 285–287), or nearby supernovas—and combinations thereof.

Devising a watch-list of such species dangers, constantly monitoring their changing likelihoods, and preparing flexible defenses against them would be an evolutionarily new, proactive, and powerful way of meeting challenges to our species' survival. Making that addition to Darwin's proposed way of in-

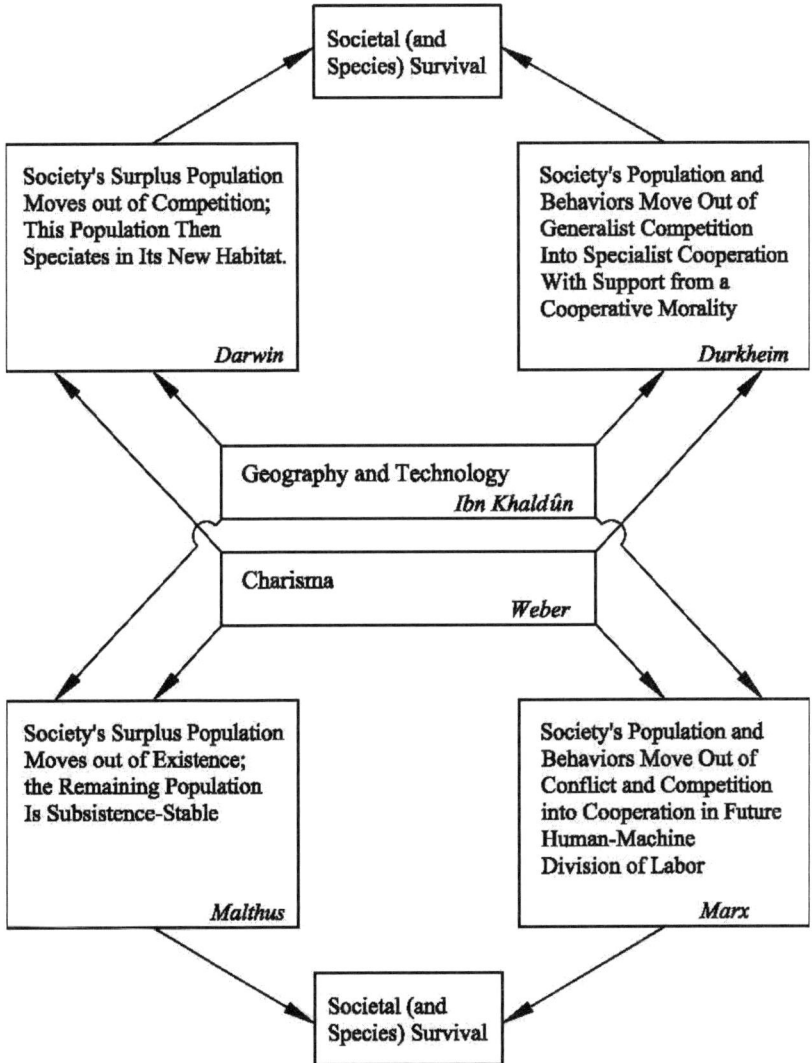

Figure 6.1. Constants Proposed by Ibn Khaldûn and Weber, and Variable Mechanisms Proposed by Malthus, Darwin, Durkheim, and Marx, for Human Societal (and Species) Survival

dividual organismic, blindly reactive, natural selection, however, requires resolving a pivotal philosophical division among sociological (and other) theorists—namely, their difference of attitude toward causal determinism and causal probabilism.[2]

This brings us to the final big issue to which this little book is addressed.

## Causal Determinism versus Causal Probabilism

In a word, *causal determinism* claims that alternatives and substitutes can never exist; that there is, and can be, one and only one possible course which everything must follow and so is following.[3] *Causal probabilism*, however, claims that at any given time and place there exist indeterminately many, variably likely, alternative causes that yield measurably the same effects, and also that there exist indeterminately many, variably likely, alternative and combinable effects that are produced by measurably the same causes.

Among the theorists covered in this book, Ibn Khaldûn is the earliest sociological determinist—a determinism expressed in his forecast that whatever rises *must* fall. Later, Auguste Comte (1798–1857), too, embraces determinism: "the progressive march of civilization follows a natural and unavoidable course"; the "main historic epochs [of the sciences] . . . through the theological and metaphysical into the positive stage . . . are rigorously determined" (1975, 39, 41). Marx, too, insists again and again on determinism: "division into classes . . . *will* be swept away by the complete development of modern productive forces" (1969, 3:147–48; see also 2:88–89); "the feudal relations of property . . . *had* to be burst asunder" (1969, 1:113); "the bourgeois period of history *has* to create the material basis of the new world"; "consciousness is something that the world *must* acquire, like it or not" (1978, 663).

But it is Durkheim who most fully exemplifies deep and unresolved *ambivalence* toward determinism and probabilism. On the one hand Durkheim tells us, deterministically, that "if a mode of behavior existing outside the consciousnesses of individuals becomes general, it can *only* do so by exerting pressure on them" (1982, 57); that "it is *inconceivable* that the same effect could be sometimes due now to one cause, now to another, according to the circumstances, unless fundamentally the two causes were but one" (1995, 418; see also 1951, 146); that "If all hearts beat in unison . . . it is because *one and the same force is propelling them in the same direction*" (1982a, 56), because "to the *same effect* there always corresponds the *same cause*" (1982a, 150, italics changed; see also 80–81, 148–149; 1995, 249); and, most explicitly, that "sociology could not emerge until the idea of *determinism* . . . was finally extended to the social order" (1960, 376).[4]

On the other hand, and without so much as acknowledging any of the above clearly deterministic declarations, Durkheim makes several unequivocal statements that substitute probabilism for those declarations: "to arrive at the same goal," he says, "*many different routes* can be, and in reality are, followed" (1982a, 122–123); "just as a single [religious] rite can serve several ends, *several rites can be used interchangeably to bring about the same end*" (1995, 390); "the term 'role' or 'function' . . . in no way prejudges the question of . . . how [the implied relationship between cause and effect] has been established . . . *whether it arises from some intended and preconceived adaptation or from adjustment after the event*" (1984, 11); both mechanical and organic solidarity "lead to the *same aim, but by opposing routes*" (1984, 330; see 1986, 393; also 1995, 412,

417); his task is to "discover the rational *substitutes* for those religious notions that for a long time have served as the vehicle for the most essential moral ideas" (1973, 9; see also 1995, 429, 431); and "an *identical* system of behavior may be adjustable to . . . *many different ends* without altering its nature"; that "there are . . . cases where *a practice or a social institution changes its functions* without for this reason changing its nature"; "it is a proposition true in sociology as in biology, that . . . while staying *the same [an organ] can serve different ends*"; and that "*several rites can be used interchangeably to bring about the same end*" (1951, 43; 1982a, 120, 121; 1995, 390; see also 1978, 65, 217; 1974, 30; 1982a, 47).

Indeed, the probabilistic side may come out in Durkheim's work most clearly when he identifies not just *one* causal path that leads individuals to commit suicide but *four* alternative, variously combinable, causal paths that can lead them to this same act (see chapter 2).

Admittedly, Durkheim defends this nondeterministic, probabilistic, position with the deterministic assertion that "*only in so far as the effective causes differ can there be different types of suicide*" (1951, 146; see the quotation from 1982a, 150, above; cf. Gane 2000). He also asserts, deterministically, that in statistical rates—of suicide, for example—"the [many different] *individual* circumstances which may have played some part in producing the phenomenon *cancel each other out*" (1982a, 55), leaving only the *sociocultural* circumstances that produced it—thereby contradicting his own claim that a rate "in no way prejudges the question of . . . how [it] has been established"—which implies that the same rate can be causally established in different ways.

In short, Durkheim seems, perhaps unknown to himself, torn between determinism and probabilism.

The choice is absolutely crucial for sociocultural policy-making. Determinism permits policies that opt only among speeds along the single possible track toward any given destination (Comte claims that "the progress of the [human] race must be considered susceptible of modification *only with regard to its speed*, and without any reversal in the order of development of any interval of any importance being overleaped" [1975, 236]). Probabilism, however, tells us that in addition to *speed* differences along one and only one track, it is also possible to choose among different *tracks* and so among different kinds and amounts of *costs* to different groups of clients, to reach a given destination[5]—and that it is also possible to choose *different destinations* which can be reached by following different paths from the same starting-point.

Weber's "ethic of responsibility," with its provision of choice among degrees of causal *efficiency* (each degree achievable in different ways) depends on the existence of such alternative possibilities and so is probabilistic—while his "ethic of ultimate ends" is deterministic and concerned only with maximizing the *effectiveness* of reaching a given goal (analogous to Comte's "speed") regardless of efficiency.

## *Many Roads Lead to Rome (Equifinality)*

It is, then, Durkheim-determinist who is speaking when we read that "if all hearts beat in unison . . . it is because *one and the same force* is propelling them in the same direction." But it is Durkheim-probabilist who tells us, with no less certainty, that "to arrive at the same goal, *many different routes can be, and in reality are, followed.*"[6]

Differences in causal processes that produce the same effects have been called "equifinality" (von Bertalanffy 1956;

Heider 1958; Braithwaite 1960), and more recently Kauffman relies on the idea (without naming it) when he says the ultimate question for biology is "what are the *alternative bases* for self-reproducing molecular systems [including life] here and anywhere in the cosmos?" (2000, 15).[7] Equifinality, then, is the basic causal model behind such folk-sayings as "All rivers run to the sea"; "All roads lead to Rome"; "All fates become one fate"; and "There is more than one way to skin a cat."[8] Equifinality, in short, is half of why we say "correlation is not causation." The other half is equi-initiality.

## *Many Roads Lead from Rome (Equi-Initiality)*

The basic idea of equifinality is exemplified when we say that matters have come to a "crisis," a "turning point," a "fork in the road," a "divergence in a wood"—all of which mean that things may proceed from some single arbitrary starting point toward many alternative end-points. In short, not only may there be *alternative causes* of the same effect (equifinality) as discussed above; there may also be *alternative effects* of the same cause (equi-initiality). Weber exemplifies the latter view as well when he tells us "action that is 'identical' in its meaning relationship occasionally takes what is, in the final effect, a radically varying course" (1981, 156).

We called this logical partner of equifinality *"equi-initiality."* (It has already been somewhat misleadingly named "multifinality" (Buckley 1967, 60)—we say "somewhat misleadingly," because *"multi*finality" implicitly includes, indiscriminately, both multiple *contributory* effects and multiple *alternative* effects without explaining that the latter is a special case of the former.) By embracing both equifinality and equi-initiality, we intend to adopt the hypotheses that "for want of a nail the shoe [*can* be] lost; For want of a shoe the horse [*can* be] lost; For want of a horse the rider [*can* be] lost; For want of a rider the battle [*can* be] lost; For want of a battle the kingdom [*can* be] lost"—which is to say that any one of these steps, and even the entire sequence, *can* happen, but the entire sequence is *vanishingly likely* to do so (see Knobe et al. 2006, 60).[9]

We fully accept, therefore, Weber's many statements (they appear to be unique in classical sociological theory) of probabilism—that is, both equifinality and equi-initiality. "The social relationship," Weber says, "consists entirely and exclusively in the existence of a *probability* that there will be a meaningful course of action"; "The same result may be reached from [different] starting-points" (1978, 26–27, 454); "processes of action which seem to an observer to be the same or similar may fit into exceedingly various complexes of motive in the case of the actual actor" (1978, 10); "behavior that is identical in its external course and result can be based on the most varied constellations of motives, and the most plausible motive may not be the one that came into play" (1981, 151); "the very 'need' to eat . . . may be essentially conditioned by various effective circumstances operating as 'stimuli'—for example, a physically empty stomach or . . . merely habituation to eating at particular hours of the day" (1975b, 29, italics removed); "common customs may have diverse origins"; "the most diverse reasons can lead to a 'No' [in a plebiscite]"; "the subjective meaning need not necessarily be the same for all the parties who are mutually oriented in a given social relationship"; "orientation to the situation in terms of the pure self-interest of the individual and of the others to whom he is related can bring about results comparable to those which imposed norms prescribe" (1978, 394, 1455, 27, 30); and that "'power' is the probability that one actor within a social relationship will be in a position to carry out his own will despite resistance, regardless of the basis on which this probability rests" (1978, 53).[10]

## A Concluding Short-Term Species Survival Proposal

On the basis of the entire argument presented in this book, we propose that training in simulative computer programming—aimed at probabilistically *forecasting* various threats to human sociocultural and species survival and at planfully (and, again, probabilistically) *preparing* alternative ways of meeting those threats—should become a required part of graduate training in sociology.[11]

# APPENDIX

# THREE CRITICAL DISAGREEMENTS ABOUT DURKHEIM'S THEORY

## 1. Durkheim's Human Sociocultural Self-Maintenance Theory

Durkheim's leading theoretical hypothesis that human sociocultural phenomena are self-maintaining does not seem to have registered on all his readers (see Alpert 1939; Hinkle 1960, 289). For example, Berger and Luckmann say nothing about sociocultural self-maintenance but claim instead that "consider social facts as *things* is Durkheims' 'marching order' for sociology" (1967, 17, 18; see also Pope 1976, 187–204; Lukes 1982, 2; Jones 1999). And indeed, Durkheim does say that "the proposition . . . that social facts must be treated as things . . . is at the very basis of our method" (note: Durkheim says our "*method*," not our *theory*), and then he tells us that "a thing is any object of knowledge which . . . [we can only understand by] *observation and experimentation*" (1982a, 35–36)—that is, by the scientific method.

So it does seem fair to say that "treat social facts as things" is Durkheim's general *methodological* "marching order" for sociology; it tells us *how* to look at phenomena—that is, as empirical, sensually verifiable, data (rather than as personally speculative, imaginative, abstractions). The proposition that human sociocultural phenomena are *self-maintaining* is, however, a general *theoretical* "marching order"; it tells us *what* to look for in phenomena—namely, the *mechanisms* through which those phenomena maintain themselves.

Parsons puts the self-maintenance proposition a little differently, and less explicitly: "it was the problem of the *integration* of the social system, of what holds societies together, which was the most persistent preoccupation of Durkheim's career" (1960, 118, see also 150; 1960, 150–151)—without stating Durkheim's key hypothesis that human societies *hold themselves* together both social structurally and culture structurally.

Jonathan Turner et al. claim that "Durkheim's . . . theoretical work revolved around *one* fundamental question: What is the basis for integration and solidarity in human societies?" (2002, 330)—overlooking that Durkheim claims the *two* factors are *different* in character and have *different* explanatory and predictive bases.

Gane argues that "Durkheim's basic theory developed and *changed* over the course of his career. . . . In the earlier writings he held that primitive societies were characterized by similitudes and passions, while the advanced societies [were characterized] by individualism and calm restraint. . . . He later revised this view *completely*" (2001, 83).

Emirbayer claims that Durkheim "provides an illuminating and comprehensive perspective upon civil society . . . [while he also] gives us the beginnings of a theory of relational social realism" (1996, 125), but without making clear the nature of "civil society" or "relational social realism."

Alexander says that "What Durkheim's science 'discovered' . . . was the importance of the very social facts his theory presupposed, namely, the importance of morality" (1982, 303), but he does not state Durkheim's criterion of that "importance" (i.e., human sociocultural self-maintenance). In addition, Alexander overlooks social structural "integration" as a "social fact" that is of equal importance to "morality" in Durkheim's theory.

Other commentators, however, come closer than the above to what we ourselves regard as the sociocultural self-maintenance theoretical mark: Merton seems right to define biological "function" as referring "to the 'vital or organic processes [inside the organism] considered in the respects in which they contribute to the *maintenance of [that] organism*'"—thus almost defining "functional analysis" as what we are calling self-maintenance analysis (we say "almost" because Merton does not say "and vice-versa," which would make the self-maintaining causal loop explicit)—and he gives Durkheim only brief citations as having "adopted a functional orientation throughout his work" (1957, 61; see also 21, 29), without stating explicitly the various ways that that orientation appears in Durkheim's work.

Duncan may have the sociocultural self-maintenance proposition vaguely in mind when he says that to Durkheim "society functions through symbols" (1960, 101—except that he does not specify that the "symbols" in question are, in Durkheim's perspective, made by the "society" in question) and so self-mediates that society's self-maintenance.

Pierce seems almost sure to have sociocultural self-maintenance in mind when he refers to Durkheim having a focus on the "*self-realization* of society" (1960, 165), as does Cormack when she claims Durkheim sees "an incessant and *circular movement* between the human manufacture of social realities, and the group's particular responses or relations to these realities," and, of course, when she quotes Durkheim's own claim that "a society can . . . *recreate itself*" (1996, 96, 97).

Pope says that "above all, Durkheim wanted to generate a strictly sociological explanation" (1976, 11) but does not specify what "a strictly sociological explanation" would be—although exploring the sociocultural self-maintenance hypothesis seems a reasonable definition. Tiryakian clearly alludes to sociocultural self-maintenance in Durkheim's theory when he says "society is both *the object and the source* of moral action," but oddly that idea does not figure at all in his enumeration of Durkheim's "three fundamental presuppositions of sociology" (1962, 27; cf. 14).

Gerstein rightly refers to Durkheim's "two-way street between individual and society" (1983, 249; cf. TenHouten 1998, 409), but he does not identify the self-maintenance of *society* (not of the *individual*) as the principal explanandum of Durkheim's theory. Tekla and Pope rightly claim that "the ultimate goal of [Durkheim's] sociological explanation [is] identifying and analyzing the social forces that cause social effects" (1985, 78), but they turn aside from this self-maintenance conclusion by asserting that "the *force* imagery constitutes the integrating element in Durkheim's thought" (1985, 86; see also 75, 78). Collins calls "the Durkheimian tradition . . . the core tradition of sociology," but whatever may be his reasons for claiming 'coreness'—which are not altogether clear to us (see 1994, 181, 183), those reasons do not appear to include sociocultural self-maintenance.

Nisbet rightly says that to Durkheim "the task of the social investigator has only begun when he distinguishes the efficient causes of any social phenomenon and traces its history; from this he must go on to determine the function of the phenomenon in the system or order of which it is a part. And the function of a social fact . . . must always be sought in the [causal] relation of the fact to some social end" (1965, 31). Oddly, however, that "task" does not figure in Nisbet's list of "five [crucial] perspectives in Durkheim's thought" (see 1965, 31).

Neither does sociocultural self-maintenance figure in Brian S. Turner's "five themes," which he says Durkheim developed (1992, xviii). Traugott does not mention sociocultural self-maintenance among the "unifying themes" of the selections from Durkheim's work that he translates and edits (1978b, 1); nor do Fenton et al. mention it among what they regard as the "three main elements of Durkheim's theories" (1984, 222–231); nor does Gane include it among the four prescriptions he finds in *The Rules of Sociological Method* (2000, 23–24; see also 1994).

Blau, too, says that "Durkheim . . . emphasized that social facts must be explained in terms of other social facts," but he then goes on to claim that "the study of social facts ... cannot be carried out by analyzing a sample of individuals but requires comparisons of societies or other collectivities" (1989, 49)—a claim that somehow ignores Durkheim's explicitly saying that "social facts . . . consist of manners of acting, thinking and feeling external to the individual, which are invested with a coercive power by virtue of which they exercise control *over [that individual]*" with the consequence that such control can *only* be analyzed if we have a sample of individuals.

Susan Stedman Jones says society, in Durkheim's view, is "an irreducible, independent reality" (2001, 149), but she explicates none of these terms—especially since Durkheim did indeed reduce society to dependency on a multiplicity of "social facts."

Rawls seems mindful of sociocultural self-maintenance—although her analysis is largely limited to *The Elementary Forms of Religious Life*—when she says to Durkheim that "the primary purpose [contrast Durkheim 1982a, 120, 123 on "purpose"] of religion is to provide the enacted practices necessary to produce the categories [of the understanding]" and that "all societies will have the categories, according to Durkheim, because, if they cannot produce the categories, they cannot exist as societies" (1996, 462; see also 446–452)—although Durkheim does not himself draw the latter conclusion. Rawls's view of exactly *how* "totemic rituals . . . give rise to the category of causality," however, is that "the causal efficacy of the ritual is *perceived directly as a feeling of moral unity* [among the participants]" (1996, 450)—a telepathy-implying claim which we (and eventually Durkheim himself) reject.

Giddens tells us that "according to Durkheim, the object of sociology is to construct theories about *human conduct*" (1979, 138), but this blurs Durkheim's more closely targeted concern (except in *Suicide*, as discussed in chapter 2) with specifically human *sociocultural* conduct and with showing how that conduct *maintains* itself.

Traugott claims that to Durkheim, "sociology's distinctive task is to demonstrate *how individual behavior is . . . the product of social forces*" (1978b, 10; see also Bueno de Mesquita et al. 2002, 270), without including any reference to the sociocultural self-maintenance hypothesis and therefore to the feedback problem of how social forces are produced by individual behavior.

## 2. Durkheim's Inconsistencies

The details of the many inconsistencies in Durkheim's theory cited in chapter 2 seem to have been passed over without direct and specific comment in the past. One guesses, however, that Lukes has some of these inconsistencies in mind when he refers to Durkheim's extremist diction as a "style" that "tends to *caricature* his thought" (1975, 4; see also 1990, 2:338–339; Bellah 1959, 452; Nisbet 1965, 36–38; Barnes 1990, 2:72; Cormack

1996, 89, 93–94)—overlooking that (1) a given thought can be "caricatured" in a large number of ways, none of which Lukes specifies or exemplifies; and (2) that we can never know what Durkheim's (or anyone else's) thought *really* was (see Gilbert 1994, 92), unless we accept telepathy.

Fields has referred to "rhetorical leaps" in Durkheim's argument, which she says one should notice *not* in order "to show where he fell short as a systematic thinker; [but] to amplify his voice and hear him better" (Fields 1995, xxi, xxii)—though she does not make clear either why one should not do both, or how we may know that the amplified voice we hear is truly Durkheim's voice and not our own.

To us it has often seemed as though Durkheim were recording his ideas almost stenographically—without giving them a self-critical backward (or forward) looking editing that all ideas deserve. Fauconnet's comment, that after writing out "in extenso" his lectures on moral education that were first given "at the Sorbonne in 1902–3, Durkheim simply repeated them "in 1906–7, without change or editing" (1973, v), seems relevant here; as does Nisbet's summary judgment that *The Division of Labor* "is a kind of palimpsest" (1965, 36). Not dissimilarly, Alexander speaks of Durkheim's "constant back-and-forth movement between aggressive assertion and just as aggressive denial" (1982, 231).

On the other hand, in noticeable contrast with the above criticisms of Durkheim's theory, Bryan S. Turner claims that Durkheim's arguments are "*invariably* logical and clear" (1992, xiii), and Traugott says that Durkheim's "thought is *thoroughly* disciplined" and that his "arguments *flow logically* from one point to the next"; and "his style remains *consistent* over three decades of intellectual development" (1978, ix). But the same Traugott then charges Durkheim with "amusing contortions"; with managing "only loosely to resolve" certain "contradictions" in his work; with being "far from consistent in applying [a particular] tenet"; and with "wavering" between two views of something, so that "we are forced to choose between what [he] says and what he does" (1978b, 4, 7, 9, 13). A "style . . . consistent over three decades"?

## 3. Social Structure and Culture Structure in Durkheim's Theory

It should be emphasized that our claim that Durkheim's theory focuses, throughout his work, on *two* interacting types of sociocultural behavior mechanisms—namely, social structure and culture structure—departs from the much more usual commentators' claim that Durkheim focuses on only *one* such mechanism, namely, culture structure (although no one but ourselves calls it that).

Parsons, for example, asserts that Durkheim regarded "the aim of sociology as that of studying the systems of *value ideas in themselves*" (1949, 446 italics changed—and not in their *consequences?*); and then, more surprisingly, that Durkheim "does *not* mean that society is a 'material' thing. . . . It is not only *not material*, but *'psychic'*" (1949, 356; see also 357; 1960, 121–122). Serving up a similar surprise, Giddens says that to Durkheim "an individual [organism] is *not a body*" (1979, 5)—without explaining how a not-body can commit suicide. Naegele says that "Durkheim dignifies society as a *moral* phenomenon that stands stubbornly *beside nature*" (1958, 581) in no less stubborn disregard of Durkheim's reference to a "science of morality . . . [that] attempts to study moral maxims and beliefs as *natural* phenomena" (1978, 63; see also 220–221). Bellah, too, sees Durkheim as focusing exclusively on "the *moral or normative* order of society" (1973, xxiii), as do Ritzer and Bell:

"At the most general level, Durkheim was a sociologist of *morality*" (1981, 972; but see 978ff).

Not dissimilarly, Bottomore and Nisbet tell us that "the overriding objective [of *The Division of Labor*] was to demonstrate the evolutionary reality and importance of the two great types of *solidarity*: 'mechanical' and 'organic'" (1978, 566) overlooking Durkheim's treatment of "segmentary" and "organized" social structure, and Fenton et al. are equally exclusive when they say that in *The Division of Labor* what Durkheim "saw to be the critical issue [was] social *solidarity*" (1984, 18). Tiryakian, too, argues that "Durkheim viewed [social science] as investigating scientifically the *normative* infrastructure of human society" (1978, 189; see also 217, 222). Traugott says that "the core of [Durkheim's] sociology [is] the explication of social *solidarity*" (1978b, 9; see also 38). Robert Alun Jones, too, says that "Durkheim's central explanatory hypothesis [is] that when social conditions [*sic*] fail to provide people with the necessary *social goals and/or rules* . . . their socio-psychological health is impaired and the most vulnerable among them commit suicide" (1986, 114)—thereby overlooking Durkheim's finding in *Suicide* that "social conditions" that fail to provide people with the necessary *social structural interactions* ("integration") can have exactly the same suicidal tendency. Willer et al. also see Durkheim focusing on culture structure (i.e., *shared ideas of "legitimacy"* [see 2002, 131–135]) alone, as does Susan Stedman Jones: "The initial question of *De la division du travail social* [is] the relation between individual *personality and social solidarity*," and "A self-referentiality of *belief* systems lies at the center of the logic of social reality [according to Durkheim]" (2001:111, 216; see also 217). Cormack argues that Durkheim made "sociology's first clear attempt to understand *representation* [that is, mental imaging] as the fundamental element of social life" (1996, 99)—thereby derogating Durkheim's attention to social structure as an equally "fundamental element of social life."

We, however, hold with Merton when he tells us that in Durkheim's theory "the source of social life . . . is *twofold . . . consciousness* and the division of social *labor*" (1934/1998, 373); with Lukes's claim that Durkheim "always remained alive to the *interaction* between social structure and [cultural] consciousness" (1975, 236); and with Collins when he describes Durkheim's "central model . . . [as] the generation of *moral solidarity* by structural arrangements of *social interaction*" (1988, 124)—despite Collins's omitting the self-maintaining *interaction* between these mechanisms—such that "moral solidarity" sustains "[social] structural arrangements," and so on, back and forth.

# Notes

## Chapter 1. Introduction

¹ Such factors take on prime importance, of course, when our interest is in the theories as phenomena to be explained—for example, in their history or sociology.

² Kauffman's "perhaps a thousandth" phrase means that the evolution of life on Earth has been no carefree stroll along Eden-like garden paths. (Incidentally, Stoeckle and Hebert tell us that "scientists [have described] some 1.7 million species" but go on to cite Edward O. Wilson (no printed source given) to the effect that "despite 250 years of effort we do not know, even to the nearest order of magnitude, how many species live on Earth [2008, 83, 86]). Instead, the career of Earthly life has been a tough, often losing, struggle to leave progeny against a succession of small and large extinctions most of whose causes are still not understood. The five largest of these extinctions occurred about 440 million, 370 million, 250 million, 200 million, and 65 million years ago. It is estimated that the largest of them all, the middle one, called "Permian-Triassic," drove our planet back nearly to its original lifelessness by terminating at least 90 percent of all the then-living species and more than 99 percent of all the then-living individual organisms (see Benton 2003, 17, 124, 175, 250). So far, however, terrestrial life as a whole has somehow survived the ravages of these and many smaller scythe-sweeps (see Benton 2003, 302, 303)—although Homo sapiens is currently mowing life down again by destroying other species' ecosystems (see Sample 2006).

³ Ants have been sociocultural for more than 50 million years (see Hölldobler and Wilson 1990, 27-29). Caution, stimulated partly by those authors' remark that "there may well be important communicative signals and social phenomena [among ants] awaiting discov-

ery" (1990, 295), leads us to use the generic term "sociocultural" here). Homo sapiens has existed and seems to have been sociocultural for only 200,000 years or so (see Ayala 1995, 1935; Klein 1989, 100).

⁴ See Angier (2008). I think it was an Arthur Clarke short story that gave me this idea, but I have forgotten its title.

⁵ See, among many others, Bosse and Treur (2006); Duong and Grefenstette (2005); Lim, Metzler, and Bar-Yam (2007); Moss and Edmonds (2005); and Moody, McFarland, and Bender-deMoll (2005).

⁶ Having thus stated our opinion of Durkheim's sociocultural self-maintenance theory as the core of all sociological theories, however, we can hardly overlook Homans's scornful groan, " 'Who cares what old Durkheim said?' " (quoted in Tilly 1981, 106)—a question that might be raised about every old theorist examined here and newer ones too. We do care what Durkheim said, though, not because we believe that his (or Malthus's, Darwin's, Marx's, Weber's, Ibn Khaldûn's, or anyone's, so far) propositions or theories are necessarily valid and reliable as whole complexities but because Durkheim's hypothesis of *sociocultural self-maintenance* still plays, and will probably long continue to play, a central role in sociological (as in other scientific) formulations no matter how complex.

⁷ Durkheim is not unaware of technological factors in human societies, for he goes to the extreme of saying "it is not true that society is made up only of individuals; [society] also includes material things. . . . For instance, a definite type of *architecture* is a social phenomenon. . . . It is the same with the avenues of communication and transportation, with the instruments and machines used in industry or private life" (1951, 313-314). We, however, see such phenomena as nonsociocultural products of sociocultural phenomena which become instruments for the latter's self-maintenance.

⁸ See Merton (1957, 162); Kroeber and Parsons (1958, 583); Parsons 1961 (33–34); cf. Burt (1992, 11); Ritzer and Bell (1981, 967); Emirbayer (1996, 110).

⁹ Merton says nothing about intended and unrecognized, or unintended and recognized, functions, but Cohen's "Law of Action asserts that it is difficult to do just what you *intended* to do" (1995, 369), clearly implying that one may do things without intending to do them.

¹⁰ Shubin applies the "participant-throughout system" idea to *organismic* systems whose participants are individual *cells* when he tells his reader, "You are the same individual you were seven years ago, even though virtually every one of your skin cells is now different: the ones you had back then are dead and gone, replaced by new ones" (2008, 118).

¹¹ For Marx's view of the public display of personal wealth and the honor and self-confidence with which onlookers in the society reward such displays, see (1967, 594), and for Veblen's view of this matter see (1979, 25–34). Neither of these theorists, however, refers to what we regard as the specialized relationship between an individual's honor and self-confidence, on the one hand, and membership in the *religious* organizations of his/her society, on the other.

¹² All four of these types of participant-organizing organizations—"political, economic and scientific . . . [and] religious" are mentioned together by Durkheim (1984, 119) but he is not consistent about that enumeration (cf., for example, 1984, xliv, 209). Merton identifies the same four, and says every participant in a given society has statuses in them all: "The same individuals have multiple social statuses and roles [in the] scientific and religious and economic and political [organizations of a society]. This fundamental linkage in social structure in itself makes for some interplay between otherwise distinct institutional [sic] spheres even when they are segregated into seemingly autonomous departments of life" (1973, 175; see also 1957, 369–370). The idea that these four types of organizations com-

prise a single participant-organizing institution is, however, unique to the present discussion.

[13] On the inevitability of some such restraint, Cohen tells us that "to believe that no ceiling to population size or carrying capacity is in prospect you have to believe that *nothing* will stop a sufficient proportion of additional people from increasing the Earth's carrying capacity by more than, or at least as much as, they consume" (1995, 445).

[14] Malthus makes no mention of Jonathan Swift's *A Modest Proposal* (1729) as proposing a super-efficient positive check on population size combined with an increase in subsistence production. Ibn Khaldûn argues that everything that rises also sets: "There is overpopulation at the end of dynasties, and pestilences and famines frequently occur then. . . . [At] the beginning, dynasties are inevitably kind in the exercise of their power and just in their administration. . . . A kind and benevolent ruler serves as an incentive to the subjects and gives them energy for cultural activities. (Civilization) becomes abundant, and procreation vigorous. . . . [However, after two generations of a dynasty's rule], there will be coercion of the subjects and bad government [and] famines and pestilences become numerous" (1958, 2:135–136). Darwin almost repeats Malthus when he says "each species tends to increase inordinately, and . . . some check is always in action, yet seldom perceived by us" (1968, 325).

[15] Note that Malthus limits his view to the evolving consequences of the distribution of *wealth* ("poverty" or "riches") without considering the similar distributions of power, honor and self-confidence, and knowledge and know-how.

[16] Darwin tells us he is interested only in the *self-maintenance*—via migration and speciation—of life, not its origin and certainly not its termination (which he doesn't mention at all) "I have nothing to do with the origin ... of life itself," he says. "We are concerned only with [life's] diversities" (1968, 234; also 161, 197, 219).

## Chapter 2. Durkheim's Core Sociological Theory

¹ Merton says, "A radical sociologism seemed to Durkheim to be the one way of maintaining the autonomy of sociology as an independent discipline, and it is to this dominant preoccupation that many of his conceptions are due" (1934/1998, 373). And although Merton neither defines "radical sociologism" nor states the "many . . . conceptions" in question, it seems a fair guess that Durkheim's view of human sociocultural phenomena as strictly autonomous is what Merton has in mind (see also Merton 1973, 338–339; Tiryakian 1962, 11; 1978, 188; Lukes 1982, 2–3; Cormack 1996, 89; Thompson 1998, 92–93; Besnard 2000, 98; TenHouten 1998, 475).

² Durkheim, however, tells us both (1) that "*collective life did not arise from individual life*; on the contrary, it is the latter that emerged from the former" (1984, 220–221; see Simmel 1955, 140–143) and (2), without batting an eyelash, that "before society existed there could only exist individuals. It is therefore *from the individual* that emanate the ideas and needs which have determined the formation of *societies*" (1982a, 125). Marx supports Durkheim's first view when he says that "My standpoint . . . can less than any other make the individual responsible for relations whose creature he socially remains" (1967, 1:10). Durkheim also tells us that "a society . . . is, in reality, composed of a multitude of small groups or small social worlds that ... live their own lives and remain basically external to one another" (1960:418). Note that, as we now expect from Durkheim, the human individual goes unmentioned here as the universal elemental constituent of those "small groups." Simmel is more definite numerically and tells us that the "simplest structures which can still be designated as social interactions occur between *two* elements" (1950:118), but he does not acknowledge that the "elements" in question must be living organisms. For his part, Durkheim is vague about the elements' nec-

essary number: "a phenomenon," he says, "can only be collective if it is common to all members of society, or at the very least to a majority" (1982a:56), and with that last phrase unaccountably rules out the possibility of *minority* collective phenomena (and we say "unaccountably" because minority sociocultural phenomena seem implicit in almost all divisions of labor). Durkheim draws closer to Simmel's specificity, however, when he replaces proportion with absolute number, saying that "in order for a social fact to exist, *several* individuals at the very least must have interacted together" (1982a:45), but does not become more specific. Note also that Durkheim defines *sociology* in three different hierarchic ways which he himself neither reconciles nor even compares. Thus: (1) "sociology can ... be defined as the science of *institutions*, their genesis and functioning" (1982a:45; see also 1982d:245); (2) "sociology is defined as the science of *societies*" (1960a:325; see also 1973b:149); and, as above, (3) in "the exact field of sociology. . . . *several individuals* at the very least must have interacted together" (1982a:56, 45).

There is a further difference between Durkheim's and Simmel's theories in the way they use the idea of hierarchic structure. Where Durkheim proposes only one hierarchic way to incorporate individuals' behaviors into society as a whole, Simmel proposes two ways which he calls "concentric" and "juxtaposed" structures (and we would call simple and complex). Referring to the simple way, Durkheim's way, Simmel says the individual's "participation in the smallest of ... groups already implies participation in the larger groups" (1955:147), and by "implies" Simmel means to exclude any voluntary choice in that participation by the individual. This, Simmel says, "is one of the first and most direct ways in which the individual, who has begun his social existence by being affiliated with one group only, comes to participate in a number of groups" (1955:148). Referring to the complex way, Simmel says it is historically the more recently developed way. "Today," Simmel says, "someone may belong, aside from his occupational position, to a scientific association, he may sit on the board of directors of a corporation and occupy an honorific position in the city government.... In this way, the objective structure of a society provides a framework within which an individual's non-interchangeable and singular characteristics may develop and find expression" (1955:150). In other words, Simmel continues, "The mere fact of multiple group affiliations enabled the person to achieve for himself an individualized situation in which the groups had to be oriented towards the individual [to retain his or her loyalties in competition with the other groups], and concludes that "Opportunities for individuation proliferate into infinity because the same person can occupy positions of different rank in the various groups to which he belongs" (1955:151).

The essential difference between these two ways (simple and complex) of aggregating individual participants into societies seems to be that Durkheim's simple way is ascriptive and involuntary (and thus *reactive*) for the individual participant (the individual has no choice but to be a member of all the more inclusive groups), whereas Simmel's complex way is achieved and voluntary (and thus *proactive*) for the individual participant (who may choose to belong or not to belong to given more inclusive groups).

Regarding Marx's idea that human society as a whole takes on a reactive, compulsory, "class structure" throughout all its constituent subgroups from the dominance of economic organizations there, Durkheim proposes that probably compulsory "assemblies" should be formed that "include representatives of employees and employers.... because too often their interests vie with one another and are opposing" (1984:lix, see also 1992:11-13). Contrast this with Ritzer and Bell's judgment that "Durkheim *saw no inherent difference between classes*" (1981:979). Contrast also the prominence of different levels of sociocultural phenomena in Durkheim's theory with Marks's claim that Durkheim made "an early commitment to *micro*sociological levels of analysis" (1974:331), and that he thought of "society" as *people in the mass*" (1974:341)—that is, presumably, not organized into subgroups at all.

³ Durkheim does not tell us so, but he requires much more knowledge of each participant in a society that is maintained by "organic" solidarity than in a society maintained by "mechanical" solidarity. In the latter, each participant needs only know the behavior expectations that apply to himself or herself and apply those same expectations to others ("Do unto others as thou would have them do unto you"). In societies maintained by "organic" solidarity, however, each participant must know the various specialized expectations of those others toward participants occupying statuses like her/his own and "Do unto those others as they would have you do unto them." Mead says that in "play," "the individual [takes] the *attitude of the other* toward himself" (1962, 134), but he adds the complexity of Durkheim's "organic" solidarity when he says "the child who plays in a *game* must be ready to take the attitude of *everyone else* involved in that game" (1962, 151).

⁴ Durkheim was probably unaware of Marx's earlier remark (1846, but not published until 1932—see Pascal 1947, xiv–xv, xvii) that "division of labor only becomes truly such from the moment when a *division [between] material and mental labor* appears" (1969, 1:33–34). So the same words, "division of labor," carry different meanings to Marx and Durkheim. To Marx it meant mainly a division between a specialization in physical labors (implementers), on the one hand, and a specialization in psychical labors (directors), on the other. To Durkheim it meant mainly a division among specialized physical labors, with no mention of specialized psychical labors. Where Marx identifies only the indicated *single* physical-psychical dimension of the division of labor, Spencer, because he is concerned with relations both within and *among* societies (where both Marx and Durkheim are concerned almost exclusively with relations *within* societies), identi-

fies *two* cross-cutting dimensions of division of labor: "The two social types contrasted by this dimension are the *militant* and the *industrial*" (1898, 1:556; see also 519). There is also a *third,* mediating, "social type," which Spencer calls "the *distributing* system," operating between the militant and the industrial systems, which performs a *physical transportational* "carrying function between [them] . . . and between the sub-divisions of each" (1898, 1:518). Spencer calls the second dimension "regulatory" and contrasts givers-of-orders from takers-of-orders—the directors and implementers mentioned above. This dimension arises, Spencer says, not from the need within one society to organize masses of workers in one place (as Marx says), but because "everywhere the wars *between* societies originate governmental structures [because such structures] increase the efficiency of corporate action against environing societies" (1898, 1:520). There is a third, mediating, type on this dimension, too—called "*internuncial*" (1898, 1:460, 531)—and it *transmits information* between directors and implementers of the same society. Incidentally, it seems that because Durkheim is not concerned with *inter*societal relations—especially *wars* where different societies are opponents and each side's religious organizations are culture structural weapons that demonize the opponent society and sanctify its own—he has only one brief mention of "demons" that we have found, and this mention claims that "it is often difficult to distinguish [demons] from gods proper (1965:40).

⁵ Recently, Flack explicates the transition from "segmentary" division of labor and "mechanical" solidarity to "organized" division of labor and "organic" solidarity as follows: "One of the biggest challenges to structural or functional integrity of nearly all complex adaptive systems . . . is conflict . . . [which] can cause ... an evolutionary arms race in which components try to outdo one another. The outcome of an arms race is often (but not always) the evolution of concerted mechanisms for competing or for controlling the negative con-

sequences of competition. . . . The evolution of [such] regulatory mechanisms [including the invention of special signals communicating subordination, the coding of a power structure into these signals, and the invention of third-party policing] translates into increased structural complexity . . . [so that] *conflict is a complexity rachet*" (2007, 53, 54, 57; see also Shubin 2008, 136–138).

[6] The problem with the names Durkheim gives to his types of social structure and culture structure is that they are metaphoric rather than abstract and so do not readily relate to other terms in the sociological literature—including terms Durkheim himself uses in his other studies, as we shall see. For Durkheim's stated reasons for naming the divisions of labor "segmentary" and "organized," see 1984 (128, 131–133, 168); for his reasons for naming the social solidarities "mechanical" and "organic," see 1984 (61, 84–85); 1986a (100).

[7] Durkheim repeatedly confounds this conclusion when he tells us that the term "social solidarity" refers to "society" *as a whole*: "the term is used to denote a more or less organized *society* composed of *beliefs and sentiments common to all the members of the group*," and there exists another kind of "society" as a whole that comprises "a system of *different and special functions united by definite relationships*" (1984, 83); that "it is the [social structural] division of labor that is increasingly fulfilling the role that once fell to the [cultural structural] common consciousness"; and that the division of labor "is mainly what holds together social entities in the higher types of society" (1984, 123). To this, Durkheim adds that "these two societies are really one. They are two facets of one and the same reality" (1984, 83). But he reneges on this unification when he says that "society can exist *only* in and by means of *individual minds*" (1995, 211) without mentioning that he also claims society exists equally in and by means of (but not "only") individual "*bodies*." In short, Durkheim himself is neither as clear nor as consistent about the difference and the relationship between social structure and culture structure as one would like.

⁸ Contrast our titling here to what Durkheim himself tells us *The Division of Labor* is about: "This book is above all an attempt to treat the facts of *moral life* according to the methods of the positive [empirical] sciences" (1984, xxv). And the same kind of discrepancy will be found between what Durkheim himself tells us *Suicide* and *The Elementary Forms of Religious Life* are about, and what we here say these books seem to us to be about. But then the question arises: how can any commentator have the gall to question an author's own statement regarding what that author's own books are about? Our reply is that an author has only the first word, not the last word on his or her works. We are here claiming only what these books *seem to us, as readers in our own time and place*, to be about (see Besnard 2000).

⁹ Note the phrase "psychology *alone*" here; it implies that Durkheim proposes that sociology, *together with* psychology, can better explain individual suicides than can either alone.

¹⁰ See also (1973, 38, 42; 1982a, 101); cf. Bellah (1973, xxviii); Dohrenwend (1990, vol. 3); Johnson (1990, vol. 3); Ritzer and Bell (1981, 986); Tilly (1981, 102); Turner (1992, xx); Collins (1994, 184); Gane (2001, 83).

¹¹ To this, Durkheim adds that "perhaps the most powerful cause [that determines choice of suicidal instrument] is the relative *dignity* attributed by each people, and by each social group within each people, to the different sorts of death. . . . Some are considered nobler, others repel as being vulgar and degrading" (1951, 292–293). (As we shall see in chapter 4, Weber would call this "dignity" and "nobility" *positive* charisma, and degradation *negative* charisma.) See Cutright and Fernquist (2001, 80), who introduce, in effect, the positive *honor* attributed to suicide itself, by whatever means, as a culture structural factor influencing individuals to kill themselves. The mention of high buildings in the text here is a rare point in Durkheim's theory at which technology appears as an explanatory factor. His citing "the means of communication and transmission" as contributing to in-

creasing "the density of society" (1984, 203; see also 1951, 314) is another such point. That rarity, in turn, calls attention to the fact that Durkheim introduces climate, topography, and other geographical factors (he calls them "cosmic factors") only once, and only to reject them as "direct" explanations for suicide: "the direct action of cosmic factors," he says, "could not explain the monthly or seasonal variations of suicide" (1951, 121).

[12] Durkheim himself delineates the subject matter of *Suicide* as follows: "Suicide has been chosen as [this book's] subject . . . because few [subjects] are more accurately defined and because it seemed to us particularly timely. . . . [In the study of suicide] real laws are discoverable which demonstrate the possibility of sociology better than any dialectical argument. . . . [Moreover, there will emerge] from every page of this book, so to speak, the impression that the individual is dominated by a *moral* reality greater than himself: namely, collective reality" (1951, 36–37, 38). He has somehow forgotten that *Suicide* identifies an *"integrative"* (social structural) as well as "regulatory" (culture structural; moral) "reality" that dominates the individual. At least two types of theoretical interpretations of *Suicide* may be found in the commentary literature. One interpretation of them sees *Suicide* as a study of the influence of society on its individual participants, as Durkheim has just said above. A second interpretation (adopted here) sees *Suicide* as a study of the socioculturally pathological influence of society toward its own termination by inducing its participants to exit it permanently. For a statement of both interpretations, see Lukes (1975, 215 versus 194, 205).

[13] Durkheim reiterates these definitions several pages later, saying that "[beliefs] are states of *opinion* . . . [rites] are particular *modes of action*"; but four pages after that he flagrantly contradicts himself, saying that "rites are *rules* of conduct that *prescribe* how man must conduct himself with sacred things" (1995, 34, 38). Although Durkheim says, in *The Division of Labor*, that "social life is derived from a

*dual* source, the similarity of *individual* consciousnesses and the *social* division of labor" (1984, 172)—which seems clearly to contradict his (and Comte's) idea that "a social fact cannot be explained except by another social fact"—five years later he simply drops reference to physical "labor" and highlights psychical *"consciousness"* alone: "The *only* thing necessary for a society to be coherent is that its members . . . *concur in the same faith*" (1973b, 48; cf. Lukes 1975, 229–244; Alexander 1982, 214–220). "*Morality* is the indispensable minimum, that which is strictly necessary, the daily bread without which societies cannot live" (1984, 13; see also 1995, 213–214). Durkheim tells us this shift of his from *materialist plus idealist* sociocultural self-maintenance mechanisms to a purely *idealist* mechanism "was *entirely* due to the studies of religious history which I had just undertaken [in 1895]" (quoted in Lukes 1975, 237). But already in 1885 Durkheim had asserted (forgetfully from the standpoint of *The Division of Labor*) that "in fact, the members of human societies are *not attached to one another by a material link but by ideal bonds*" (1978, 94; see also 1973a, 16). One imagines that Durkheim's lifelong eagerness to avoid being associated with Marx's work ("we have *in no way* been influenced [by Marx]," quoted in Lukes 1975, 231–232; see also 1982a, 163) may have had something to do with this denial. On the other hand, Durkheim's still later (1912) claim that "a society is the most powerful collection of *physical* and moral forces that we can observe in nature" (1995, 447) suggests that his shift from materialism was not a complete one. However, Durkheim defines "religious phenomena" not as psychical "faith" alone but as including "beliefs *and [physical] rites*" and emphasizes that "every religion is made up of intellectual *conceptions* and ritual *practices*" (1995, 34, 99). Then, so that we do not miss the culture structure versus social structure distinction here (a distinction to which, as we have indicated, Durkheim himself occasionally closes his eyes), he tells us that "between these two categories of phenomena lies all that separates *thinking* from *doing*" (1995, 34; see also 44, 430; 1956, 91, 107).

[14] Durkheim says that "totemism . . . [distinguishes] three categories of [sacred] things . . . the totemic emblem, the plant or animal whose appearance that emblem imitates, and the *members of the clan*" (1995, 141); and that "*every member of the clan is supposed to carry within himself a share of the totem whose cult is the religion of the clan*" (1992, 161).

[15] Parsons, then, seems right when he claims that to Durkheim the sacred and the profane "are not distinguished . . . in terms of any intrinsic properties of the things themselves, but in terms of human *attitudes* toward them," and describes that "attitude" as a cognitive attribution of extraordinariness combined, perhaps, with positive cathexis: "Sacred things . . . are thought of as imbued with peculiar virtues, as having special powers. . . . Above all man's relations to sacred things are *not taken as an ordinary matter of course*, but always as a matter of *special* attitudes, *special* respect, *special* precautions" (1949, 411–412; see also 415–417). Against Parsons, however, one is baffled by Durkheim's own claim that "there is *nothing extraordinary about the respect* [*that the sacred*] *inspires*" (1995, 35).

[16] Simmel says that "the individual feels himself carried by the 'mood' of the mass, as if by an external force that is quite indifferent to his own subjective being and wishing" (1950, 35; see also Weber 1978, 241–245; LeBon 1960; Blumer 1946, 172–173; Parsons 1949, 435, 436, 439). In such a situation, Simmel says, a chain-reaction occurs: "the individual, by *being* carried away, *carries* away" (1950, 35)—and Durkheim himself rightly underscores the *non*telepathic, physically expressive, mechanisms of this carrying away of others (and self): "by *expressing* [their] excitement, [the individuals] also reinforce it" (1995, 218)—in themselves as well as in others.

[17] Durkheim does observe, however, that the simple society's "women and children" are *excluded* by the adult men in that society

from the "consecrated ground" on which religious ceremonies are performed (see 1995, 384; see also 1986c, 52), and so excluded from full membership in the whole society.

[18] Note the contrast between Durkheim's statement of this project as belonging to *applied* science and his emphatically *pure* science claim that "science studies . . . facts to know them, and only to know them, in an absolutely disinterested fashion. . . . Science begins at the point where knowledge, whatever it may be, is sought for itself. No doubt, the scientist knows well that his discoveries will very probably be usable. . . . But so far as he devotes himself to scientific investigation, he is *disinterested in practical consequences*. He says what is; he establishes what things are, and he stops there" (1956, 93, cf. 99, 102, 106). Durkheim also claims, apparently unaware of his self-contradiction, that sociology "can give us . . . a body of guiding ideas that may be the core of our *practice* and that sustain it" (1956, 134; consider also the obviously practical focus of *Moral Education,* discussed below).

## Chapter 3. Marx's Supplementary Theory

[1] For simplicity, we refer all views that Marx authored, whether alone or with Engels, to Marx. Only references to writings authored by Engels alone cite Engels.

[2] Comte's view is similar to Marx's and Weber's: "social phenomena must always be founded on the necessary inevitableness of the *human* organism. . . . No sociological view can therefore be admitted . . . that is contradictory to the known laws of *human* nature" (1975, 255)—although this overlooks all non-human "social phenomena."

[3] Marx may have derived his emphasis on economic organizations from having read Malthus and Darwin—both of whose works he cites (see, for example, 1967, 1:162, 213, 313, 341, 352, 372)—

insofar as they concentrated on the bearing of economic production on the growth, and migration, of a society's population.

[4] Marx overlooks here the fungus-growing—thus, subsistence-producing—ants, already known to biological science in his time, and discussed in our own time by Hölldobler and Wilson (1990, 596–608).

[5] The last (incomplete) chapter of the final volume of Marx's book, *Capital*, is entitled "Classes," and he says here only that "there are three great social groups whose members . . . live on wages, profit and ground-rent respectively, on the realization of their labor-power, their capital, and their landed property." But he immediately has second thoughts: "However, from this standpoint physicians and officials, e.g., would also constitute two classes, for they belong to two distinct social groups, the members . . . receiving their revenue from one and the same source [a source that Marx does not name]. The same would also be true of the infinite fragmentation of interest and rank into which the division of social labor splits laborers as well as capitalists and landlords . . . the latter, e.g., into owners of vineyards, farm owners, owners of forests, mine owners and owners of fisheries" (1967, 3:886). Thus does Marx's conceptualization of economic "classes," in the end, reduce toward role-differentiated *individuals*.

[6] Marx summarily dismisses religious organizations as, together with law and morality, "so many bourgeois prejudices, behind which lurk in ambush just as many bourgeois interests" (1969, 1:118). In chapter 4 we shall see Weber claim that the Protestant religious organizations oriented their members' different activities in the capitalistic economic organizations of European societies toward peacefully *cooperative* roles there—rather than toward the "class *struggles*" that Marx claimed characterized them.

[7] Engels goes on to claim that Marx's discovery was "that mankind must first of all eat, drink, have shelter and clothing, before it can pursue politics, science, art, religion, etc.: that therefore the pro-

duction of the immediate material means of subsistence and consequently the degree of economic attained by a given people or during a given epoch form the foundation upon which the state institutions, the legal conceptions, art, and even the ideas on religion, of the people concerned have been evolved, and in the light of which they must, therefore, be explained, instead of vice-versa" (1969, 3:162). To us, however, a more apt description of Marx's thesis—as we shall try to make clear below—centers on his forecasting the still possible reversal of relationship between "instruments of labor" and "human labor-power."

[8] Shortly before the term "instruments of production" is introduced, there is an editorial note in the English translation that "four pages of the manuscript are missing here" (1969, 1:51), so we may be missing an important transitional discussion here.

[9] Veblen, however, warns us that "In the nature of the case, the desire for wealth can scarcely be satiated in any individual instance, and evidently a satiation of the average or general desire for wealth is out of the question. . . . [for] the struggle [for wealth] is substantially a race for *reputability* on the basis of an invidious comparison [and] no approach to a definitive attainment is possible" 1979, 33.

[10] We specify "mode of [*economic*] production" here because, in our view, all the participant-organizing organizations (e.g., political parties, religious congregations) produce different goods or services (as indicated in chapter 1) and have their own distinctive ways of producing them.

[11] See also Marx's references to "the various economic forms of society" (1967, 1:217) and to the various "specific historical form[s]" of the labor process (1967, 3:882).

[12] Regarding "raw materials," Marx says that if "subject of labor has, so to say, been filtered through previous labor," then we call it raw material; such as ore already extracted and ready for washing" (1967, 1:178). So there are two kinds of "subjects of labor": natural

geographic materials still in situ, and raw materials already extracted and processed—and "with the exception of the extractive industries . . . all branches of industry manipulate raw materials, objects already filtered through labor" (1967, 1:181).

[13] Again, "capital consists not only of means of subsistence, instruments of labor and raw materials, not only of material products" (1969, 1:160). Marx also explicitly brings in the *social structure* of economic organizations that produces those material products when he says that "all capital is divided into means of production and *living labor-power*" (1967, 1:612). Moreover, he brings in economic *culture structure* when he says "capital . . . consists just as much of *exchange values*" (1969, 1:160), because "all the products of which [capital] consists are *commodities* . . . [that is, they are] products which are exchangeable for other [products]. The particular ratio in which they are exchangeable constitutes their *exchange value* or, expressed in money, their *price*" (1969, 1:160).

[14] Note that the paragraph in which this lush passage appears is cut down, by an anonymous editor of the English translation, from about twenty-nine lines (1947, 22) to seven lines (1969, 1:34).

[15] Darwin says that "competition will generally be most severe . . . between the [living] forms which are most like each other" (1968, 324), and that implies competition will be present to some degree among all life forms, because they are all like each other in being living. Marx, however, claims that "division of labor only becomes *truly* such from the moment when a *division of material and mental labor* appears" (but one wonders whether Marx can have been thinking that the biologically reproductive division of labor between females and males was *not* a "true" one—a point on which Engels, his frequent collaborator, had his own view. "Division of labor was a pure and simple outgrowth of nature," Engels says, "it existed only between the two sexes. The men went to war, hunted, fished, provided the raw material for food and the tools necessary for these pursuits. The

women cared for the house, and prepared food and clothing; they cooked, weaved, and sewed. Each was master in his or her own field of activity: the men in the forest, the women in the house" (1969, 3:317; see also 231, 319)—with no mention of production of sperm and ovum.

[16] What Marx himself says is that "surplus-labor" is more labor than would be "sufficient to buy the average amount of [a laborer's] daily necessaries, or to maintain himself as a laboring man." Let us suppose, he says, that the labor just adequate to achieve this maintenance were "*six hours of average labor*." But "in buying the laboring power of the workman . . . the capitalist has . . . acquired the [culture structural] right to use or make that laboring power work during the *whole day or week*. . . . [The capitalist] will, therefore, make him work, say, daily, *twelve* hours. Over and above the six hours required to replace his wages . . . he will, therefore, have to work *six other hours*, which I shall call hours of *surplus labor*" (1969, 2:57, 58). And "here," Marx says, "we come to the rub"—the nub of class struggle (1969, 2:57): the employer wants the employee to work as much time without pay as possible; the worker wants to be paid as much as possible for all his or her work. It seems noteworthy that in this argument, the employer deprives the employee in *absolute* terms (that is, relative to the latter's genotypically fixed minimum subsistence needs). But suppose "when productive capital grows, the demand for labor grows; consequently, the price of labor, wages, goes up"—though only temporarily. At that point, Marx argues, a socioculturally *relative* deprivation of the working class takes over: "A house may be large or small; as long as the surrounding houses are equally small it satisfies all social demands for a dwelling. But let a palace arise beside the little house. . . . The little house shows now that its owner has only very slight or no demands to make. . . . [T]he occupant of the relatively small house will feel more and more uncomfortable, dissatisfied and cramped within its four walls. . . . Thus, al-

though the enjoyments of the worker have risen, the social satisfaction that they give has fallen in comparison with the increased enjoyments of the capitalist, which are inaccessible to the worker. . . . Our desires and pleasures spring from society," he says, and because "they are of a *social* nature, they are of a *relative* nature" (1969, 1:163; see also Veblen 1979, 85).

[17] Marx may be modifying this claim when he says that "all collisions in history have their origin . . . in the contradiction between the productive forces and the *form of intercourse*" (1947, 73; see also 74) instead of "property relations," which has a narrower reference than "form of intercourse" insofar as the latter includes *all* sociocultural behavior.

[18] Where chapter 2 found Durkheim focusing almost entirely on *intra*societal developments, Marx (and Spencer) refers to *inter*societal developments as well: "The exchange of commodities . . . first begins on the boundaries of . . . communities, at their points of contact with other similar communities, or with members of the latter. So soon, however, as products once become commodities in the external relations of a community, they also, by reaction, become so in its internal intercourse" (1967, 1:87; see also 351). In sum, Marx says, "the modern history of capital dates from the creation in the 16th century of a *world-embracing* market" (1967, 1:146).

[19] A machine-centered perspective is also conceivable in contrast with Marx's human-centered one. In the former, human society would be machines' way of making better machines. Dawkins says that "[genes] are the replicators and we are their survival machines. When we have served our purpose we are cast aside" (1976, 37).

## Chapter 4. Weber's Supplemental Theory

[1] Two further prefatory points: First, as will be seen shortly, we do not hold with Lukes's judgment that Weber's uses of the word "rational" and its cognates are "*irredeemably opaque and shifting*"

(1979, 207). Second, Mead seems directly to *oppose* our claim that meaning is an imaginative human attribution to an otherwise meaningless universe by claiming that "The meanings of things or objects are *actual inherent* properties or qualities of them; the locus of any given meaning is in the thing which, as we say, 'has it'" (1962, 122, n. 29). But by way of explication, Mead adds an incongruous point of human sociocultural reference: "If a gesture [of one human organism indicates] to another [human] organism the subsequent (or resultant) behavior of the given organism, then it has meaning" (1962, 76). This chapter revisits but does not repeat part of Wallace (1994).

[2] Freud also claims that "civilization . . . obtains mastery over the individual's dangerous desire for aggression by weakening and disarming it and by setting up an agency [called 'conscience'] within him to watch over it, like a garrison in a conquered city" (1962, 70–71). Note also that Freud claims that the instinctual unconscious (called the "Id") contains concepts of "good" as well as "evil" (see 1962, 64–69).

[3] Other interpreters seem to disagree. For example, Sayer claims that "*value* . . . [is] exactly that which gives all human life and action their meaning" and that "science, in its very rationality, undermines exactly those standpoints from which value is capable of being derived: above all religious ethics" (1991, 150)—thereby ignoring the meaning-giving quality of means, which is what Weber claims is what "technology" helps us find (see chapter 5). Bologh, too, claims that "the dilemma of modern life arises from the decline of (religious) *ethics*" (1990, 127) and points to what she calls Weber's acceptance of "the *replacement* of human values (ends) with technical bureaucratic means" (1990, 93).

[4] Weber does not explicitly define an actor's "means" or "end." We infer from his writings that they represent a cause-and-effect pair wherein a means is a humanly identified, and presumably humanly manipulable, *cause* of one or more humanly valued *effects* called

ends—whether the latter are immediate, intervening, or ultimate effects.

⁵ We would define a "definition" as any description that is accepted as a standard against which other descriptions are compared.

⁶ For some views of Weber's conceptualization of "rationality" with which this statement is at odds in one way or another, see Albrow (1990, 124, 154); Alexander (1982, 26–28, 152; 1988c, 84); Andreski (1984, 59); Beetham (1985, 68–69); Bendix (1960, 89–90); Bologh (1990, 122); Brubaker (1984, 2); Burger (1987, 215); Collins (1986b, 42–44, 62–79); Giddens (1979, 42, 44); Habermas (1971, 9); Hennis (1983, 157); Hindess (1987, 139, 142); Huff (1984, 68); Kalberg (1980, 1150; 2002, xi–lxxxi, esp. lxxix); Kellner (1985, 94, 106); Levine (1981, 10, 15); Marcuse (1971, 135); Martindale and Riedel (1958, xviii); Mommsen (1985, 252; 1987, 40); Nozick (1993, 64); Orum (1988, 397); Parkin (1982, 36); Parsons (1937, 58; 1947, 14, 16, 80); Ritzer (1992, 96, 97, 99); Sayer (1991, 114); Schluchter (1979a, 14–15); Schroeder (1992, 34–42); Segady (1987, 89, 135); Sica (1988, 171 194); Swidler (1973, 36, 39); Tenbruck (1980, 321, 326, 343); Tominaga (1989, 129); Turner et al. (1989, 196–197); Weiss (1985, 128); Wiley (1987, 13, 14); Wrong (1970, 26); Wuthnow (1987, 203; 1988, 489).

⁷ The same type of problem applies to Kalberg's "means-end rationality" and "value-rationality" translations (see 2002, xlvi–xlvii).

⁸ These remarks by Weber seem clearly to rule out Albrow's conclusion that "for [Weber] rational method and science were *identical* with each other" (1990, 154).

⁹ Regarding the *empirical* referents of the informational organizations, Weber asserts that "the [explanatory] situation is absolutely identical in such fields of knowledge as mathematics and the natural sciences . . . they all begin as hypotheses, flashes of imaginative 'intuition,' and are then 'verified' against the facts. . . . The same is true in history" (1978b, 121; see also Popper's reiteration of this point

[1961, 31–32] without referring to Weber). And regarding the *intersubjectivity* of scientific organizations, Weber says that, "even the knowledge of the most certain propositions of our theoretical sciences . . . is, like the cultivation and refinement of the conscience, a product of *culture*" (1949, 55; see also Popper 1961, 44–48).

[10] Therefore, when he also says that "the highest degree of rational understanding is attained in cases involving the meanings of logically or mathematically related propositions" (1978, 5), Weber probably means the highest degree of *formally* rational understanding. For a comparison of Simmel and Weber on this, see Atoji (1984, 68–75).

[11] Similarly, although we noted earlier Weber's claim that "all kinds" of salvation-oriented ethics are rational, and that only rules that are "capable of being expressed in numerical, calculable terms" are rational, we argue here that Weber—not having the benefit of Stevens's scale of scales—probably means that "all kinds" of salvation ethics are generically rational but that some are minimally rational in a "formal" sense, and others are maximally rational in that sense, according to the measurement scales they use.

[12] Andreski seems mistakenly critical of Weber when he says, "If by 'emotional' action we mean actions accompanied by emotion, then this attribute neither presupposes nor excludes rationality" (1984, 36), for Weber seems clearly to mean more than "accompanied by"; he means *motivated* by. Similarly, Andreski says, "Assuming that the most important goal is to survive, sticking to the old and proven ways may be the most rational course in primeval conditions" (1984, 36). But Weber means that a course of action is *non*rational (traditional) if it is taken *merely* because it is old. Why Habermas relegates "traditional action" to an undefined "residual category" (1971, 281) is not clear to us.

[13] It must be added, however, that neither affectual nor traditional nonrationality seems, in Weber's view, to be absolutely distinct

from the rationalities. Both nonrationalities may, in time, become rational as alternative possible affects and traditions, as alternative ultimate "ends," are conceptualized and then diffused in a population by "contagion" (see Weber 1978, 25, 23, 1377; Durkheim 1995, 217–220, 328–329). The reverse process also seems possible, wherein particular alternatives become charismatically endowed with affect, or become routinized into unexamined traditions, and so become increasingly nonrational. In this way, a given culture structure can evolve toward greater or lesser rationality.

[14] Against these words, it is surprising to find that some of Weber's interpreters claim he believed that "charisma is temporally bound—a social form that is limited to *pre*modern stages of social evolution and development," and "for Weber, then, pure charisma . . . can occur only under *pre*industrial social conditions" (Bradley 1987, 40); or that "according to Weber's own projection, charisma could hardly flourish in a 'disenchanted' world" (Glassman and Murvar 1984, 4); or that "in a rationalized world charismatic revolution is *impossible*" (Swatos 1984, 205).

[15] Similarly, Ibn Khaldûn says that "one cannot expect [prophets] to be able to work the wonder of achieving superiority without group feeling. . . . If someone who is on the right path were to attempt (religious reforms) in this way, his isolation would keep him from (gaining the support of) group feeling and he would perish" (1969, 127–128). Thomas and Thomas, however, say that "if men define situations as real, they [presumably, the definitions, not the situations which, if they are *not* real, have no consequences] are real in their consequences" (1928, 572).

[16] Shils says that "one of the greatest dispersions [of charisma] in history is that which has taken place in modern states, in which an attenuated charisma, more dispersed than in traditional aristocracies (where it was already more dispersed than in primitive tribes or absolute monarchies), is shared by the *total adult citizenry*" (1968, 390).

[17] Simmel also stresses charismatic exceptionality in erotic relationships: "the lovers think that there has never been a love like theirs; that nothing can be compared either to the person loved or to the feelings for that person" (1950, 406).

[18] The nature of that "tie," to Weber, is not clear. The same uncertainty of causal transmission is present in Comte's argument that "it is the formation of capital that is the true source of the great moral and mental results [often attributed] to the distribution of industrial tasks [that is, the division of labor]" (1975, 406); and in Marx's claim that the "social relations of production change, are transformed, with the change and development of the material means of production" (1969, 1:160).

[19] For Marx's view of the Protestant Reformation, see Marx (1969, 3:103–114).

[20] Weber does not stop to consider that human drive of competitiveness to make more and more money, which Veblen points out when he tells us that "the desire for wealth can scarcely be satiated in any individual instance, and evidently a satiation of the average or general desire for wealth is out of the question. However widely, or equally, or 'fairly,' it may be distributed, no general increase of the community's wealth can make any approach to satiating this need, the ground of which is the *desire of everyone to excel everyone else in the accumulation of goods*" (1979, 32).

[21] Weber says that "a distinction must be made between the theology of Calvin and *Calvinism*, and between the theological system and the necessities of pastoral care" (2002, 200)—thereby exemplifying the distinction between charisma and its routinization.

[22] Marx, as we saw in chapter 3, forecast the *robot*. Weber *almost* forecast *artificial intelligence*: "The fully developed bureaucratic apparatus compares with other forms of organization exactly as does the machine with the non-mechanical modes of production. . . . A non-living machine is mind objectified . . . [just as is] that animated

machine, the bureaucratic organization" (1978, 973, 1502; see Inbar 1979).

## Chapter 5. The Supplemental Theories of Ibn Khaldûn and Others

[1] Focusing on the culture structural motivation leading to the construction and operation of technological phenomena (and not counting serendipity), Weber defines "technology" as being culture structurally oriented "to the problem, given the end, of choosing [forecasting] the appropriate means" (1978, 67 italics removed). He does not mention the problem of given a means, how to choose an appropriate end. Bell tells us that "technology . . . is the use of scientific knowledge to specify [forecast] ways of doing things in a reproducible manner" (1973, 29) without mentioning the physically constructed "ways" themselves. This chapter revisits, but does not repeat, part of Wallace (1983).

[2] For readers unfamiliar with Ibn Khaldûn's name, we note that Lawrence, in his "Introduction to the 2005 Edition" of *The Muqaddimah: An Introduction to History*, tells us that "Arnold J. Toynbee, has called [Ibn Khaldûn's work] 'undoubtedly the greatest work of its kind that has ever yet been created by any mind in any time or place'" (2005, viii–ix, n4), and that Dawood says *The Muqaddimah* "can be regarded as the earliest attempt made by any historian to discover a pattern in the changes that occur in man's political and social organization" (Dawood 1969, ix).

[3] Spencer says "Social growth proceeds by . . . compounding and re-compounding. The primitive social group . . . never attains any considerable size by simple increase. . . . The formation of a larger society results only by the joining of such smaller societies. . . . After such compound societies are consolidated, repetition of the process on a larger scale produces doubly-compound societies; which, usually cohering but feebly, become in some cases quite coherent. . . . [The]

stages of compounding and re-compounding have to be passed through in succession. . . . [N]o great society is formed by the direct union of the smallest societies"—and this succession of compounding and re-compounding is accomplished "by conquest or by federation in *war*" (1898, 1:466, 467, 468, 555). War, however, has evolutionary limitations, Spencer claims: "Though, during barbarism and the earlier stages of civilization, war [furthers] . . . the development of those valuable powers, bodily and mental, which war brings into play; yet . . . after a certain stage of progress, instead of furthering bodily development and the development of certain mental powers, becomes a cause of retrogression during the later stages of civilization. . . . Perpetual warlike activities repress sympathy . . . they cultivate aggressiveness to the extent of making it a pleasure to inflict injury" (1961, 178, 179).

[4] Freud says "Man has . . . become a kind of prosthetic God. When he puts on all his auxiliary [technological] organs he is truly magnificent" (1962, 38–39)—a point Freud, uniquely among classical sociological theorists, applies to *psychically* auxiliary technology when he says "'The future may teach us," he says, "to exercise a direct influence, by means of particular chemical substances, on . . . *the mental apparatus*'" (quoted in Habermas 1971, 247).

[5] Compare Durkheim's similar but more generalized observation that "society . . . [is] disposed on the face of the earth in a certain fashion, dispersed in a countryside or concentrated in cities and so on. It occupies a more or less extensive territory, situated in a certain way relative to the seas and to the territories of neighboring peoples" (1978, 79; see also 1986c, 62–72; 1995, 425, 442–443).

[6] Weber tells us "the city is a relatively closed settlement, and not simply a collection of a number of separate dwellings. As a rule the houses in cities . . . are built very close to each other, today normally wall-to-wall," and on the other hand the city is "a colony so extensive that the reciprocal personal acquaintance of the inhabitants,

elsewhere characteristic of the neighborhood, is lacking" (1978, 1212).

⁷ Ellen Churchill Semple points out that "the most important geographical fact in the past history of the United States has been their location on the Atlantic opposite Europe; and the most important geographic fact in lending a distinctive character to their future history probably will be their location between the North Atlantic and the North Pacific, between the mainsprings of western and occidental civilizations and culture" (1933, 1).

## Chapter 6. Summary and Conclusion

¹ In this review, Durkheim asserts that "for our part, we arrived at [the postulate that the] substratum on which [the collective consciousness—that is, mechanical solidarity and organic solidarity] depends . . . [is] the members of society.... This postulate seems to us self-evident . . . [and] we arrived at this postulate before we had learnt of Marx, *whose influence we have in no way undergone*" (1982, 171)—who else, having read any theorist's work, would make such an absolute no-influence statement?

² For a recent discussion of probabilism (and of equifinality and equi-initiality—discussed below), see Vilenkin (2006, 106–111).

³ Knobe et al. rightly refer to "the strong form of determinism according to which nothing can possibly happen other than what actually does happen" (2006, 54). According to probabilism, however, alternatives *were* present, *are* present, and *will* (probably) continue being present to anything that actually does happen.

⁴ Durkheim asserts that "the social realm does not escape the law of universal determinism" (1978, 78). It is therefore difficult to know what Bellah can mean when he says that "Durkheim [was] never a devotee of one-way determinism" (1959, 458)—unless he is contrasting a "one-way" with some "many-way" determinism that he does not explicate, or is alluding to Durkheim's also unexplicated ambivalence

toward both determinism and probabilism. For other comments on Durkheim's remarks, see Tekla and Pope (1985, 77, 78); Lukes (1975, 32); Jones (1986, 113); Collins (1988, 109).

[5] In the deterministic view of the world, explanation and forecasting (prediction) raise exactly the same problem relative to two different time-periods (i.e., the past to the present, and the present to the future)—and that problem is to find the one and only set of conditions (Durkheim's "one and the same force") that can possibly produce a given effect regardless of time-period (see Hempel and Oppenheim 1948; Popper 1961, 252–253; Van Fraassen 1991, 41)—which implies that the universe does not change over time (but we now know, of course, that it has changed, and is changing, profoundly). Feigl defines determinism as "ideally complete and precise predictability, given the momentary conditions, the pertinent laws, and the required mathematical techniques" (see also Hempel's discussion of "Laplace's demon" [1965, 88]), and contrasts it with "statistical . . . predictability on the basis of stable frequency-ratios or according to strict laws governing frequency ratios" (1953, 411, 409, italics removed). One might say that Einstein's belief that God does not play dice with the world is deterministic, but the belief that dice play God with the world is probabilistic. Of the two, Pareto tells us that "science . . . cannot and must not accept determinism *a priori*," for "every inquiry of ours . . . is contingent, relative, yielding results that are just more or less probable" (1935, paragraphs 132 and 5). More recently, Barnett argues that "self-organizing systems [including social systems] are *not deterministic*, rather they allow for a certain degree of randomness or uncertainty in the relations among the components," and this "allows for variance in the system's trajectory such that over time the range of system states is nearly endless" (2005, 4).

[6] See, for example, Cutright and Fernquist (2001, 77), who point out that the same gender gap in suicide rates can result from a range of covariations in male and female suicide rates, each of which may

have its own causes (see also Oliver and Marwell [2002, 182]; Fararo and Skvoretz [2002, 308]), and that any of these forces could be substituted for any of the others with no effect on the gap in rates.

[7] Other implicit applications of equifinality may be found in Barrow (1988, 142–143); Blakeslee (2001); Bueno de Mesquita et al. (2002, 272, 273); Darwin (1968, 220); Feynman (1985); Greene (2004, 151); Heider (1958, 101); Heckathorn (2002, 96, 102); Holland (1998, 33–34, 36, 49–50); Ibn Khaldûn (1967, 390); Jepperson (2002, 238, 240); Kauffman (1995, 78, 100, 110); Levi-Setti (1993, 57); Merton (1957, 52); Morowitz (2002, 11, 20, 21); Oliver and Marwell (2002, 189); Shibutani (1968, 332); Simon (1965, 158; 1973, 16); von Bertalanffy (1956, 4); Wagner and Berger (2002, 46, 48, 53); Weber (1978, 27).

[8] Merton rightly refers to "the *range* of possible variation in the items which can . . . subserve a functional requirement" and says that that "range" is "not unlimited" (1957, 52, italics changed). Such a range cannot be *un*limited because that would imply that *any* variation of *any* set of *any* items could equally well serve a given functional requirement (which could then hardly be called a "requirement"). It seems fair to guess that some effects may be served by a wide range of causes (and vice-versa), others by a narrow range, down to only one particular cause and/or one particular effect—at which point we recognize determinism as a special, extremely unlikely, case of probabilism. Thus, Dawkins says that "sometimes there are two, or more, alternative [biochemical] pathways to the same useful end. . . . Either of the two alternative pathways will do the job, and it doesn't matter which one is used" (1987, 171). Robertson relies on the principle of equifinality when he says that "the world-as-a-whole could, in theory, have become the [single, global] reality which it now is in ways and along trajectories other than those which have actually obtained . . . [including] the imperial hegemony of a single nation or a 'grand alliance' between two or more dynasties

or nations; the victory of 'the universal proletariat'; the global triumph of a particular form of organized religion; the crystallization of 'the world spirit' [etc.]" (1990, 21). Pareto accepts equifinality when he says that "identical facts may be explained by an infinite number of theories—all equally true, for all reproduce the facts in their explanation" (1966, 144–145; see also Mannheim 1955, 282). Leakey and Lewin accept it when they emphasize that "similar anatomy does not always imply close evolutionary relationship . . . [for] identical anatomy may appear in two unrelated groups when they adapt to identical pressures of natural selection" (1992, 79). Chomsky uses the term "transformational grammar" to signify the systematic limits placed on equifinality in linguistic phrase structure ("*many* pairs of sentences are assigned similar or identical representations on some level" [1957, 107; see also 85–86, 90, 93]). This makes it essential to add that whether there is more than one way to skin a cat depends on how broadly or narrowly one *defines* the skinned-cat condition, and how much of various resources one is prepared to spend to achieve that condition. Thus, although Dawkins describes many cases of "convergent [biological] evolution" (for example, eyes in trilobites, octopi and humans), he also notes that "when we look *in detail* we find . . . that the convergence is not total. The different lines of evolution betray their independent origins in numerous points of detail" (1987, 94). And Barrow says that "whereas we can envisage different forms of life, based upon chemistries other than carbon or even based upon something non-chemical, only carbon-based life can evolve spontaneously" (1991, 195). Equifinality, then, does not propose that any two or more causes can produce *absolutely*—that is, *philosophically*—identical effects; we only need think of these effects as *empirically undiscriminated by some given measurement*. Infinitely precise measurement procedures might reveal infinite differences. Or they might not.

⁹ Consider a couple of other examples: "Suppose you are buying a car. . . . And suppose, for the sake of simplicity, that there are just two models to choose from. Call them A and B. . . . So what do you do? . . . You start asking your friends. And then it happens, purely by chance, that the first two or three people you talk to say that they've been driving car A. They tell you that it works fine. So you decide to buy one, too. . . . With enough lucky breaks like this, car A will come to dominate the market. . . . In fact . . . with a few lucky breaks either way in the beginning, this kind of process can produce any outcome at all" (Waldrop 1992, 45–46). Or, similarly, "who could have imagined that . . . many of the giants of European classical music—Schoenberg, Stravinsky, Rachmaninoff and Otto Klemperer (to say nothing of Mann and Adorno)—would end up living on each other's doorsteps in Los Angeles?" (Dyer 2007, 9). Finally, and more consequentially, Canup tells us that "were it not for the moon, the influence of the giant planets in our system would cause . . . the angle between the Earth's equator and the plane of its orbit . . . to vary wildly. . . . Such variation would probably cause extreme climatic changes that would render the planet uninhabitable. Thus having a large moon may be one of the key characteristics necessary for a habitable Earth-like planet" (1999, 6; see also Ward and Brownlee 2000, 221–242).

¹⁰ See also Marx (1969, 1:108–109); Bottomore (1981, 910); Heckathorn (2002, 83); Goldstone (2002, 207); Richardson (2002, 3); Wheeler (1998, 269); Wolfram (2002, 1196–1197).

¹¹ Apparently with a similar thought in mind, Diamond says that "the challenge now is to develop human history as a science, on a par with acknowledged historical sciences such as astronomy, geology, and evolutionary biology" (1999, 408)—but he does not mention empirically based forecasting and planned preparation for likely future events as being essential applied goals of those and all empirical sciences.

## References

Albrow, Martin. 1990. *Max Weber's Construction of Social Theory*. Houndmills: Macmillan.
Alexander, Jeffrey C. 1982. *The Antinomies of Classical Thought: Marx and Durkheim*. Berkeley: University of California Press.
———. 1988. *Durkheimian Sociology: Cultural Studies*. New York: Cambridge University Press.
Alpert, Harry. 1939. "Explaining the Social Socially." *Social Forces*, vol. 17, no. 3 (March): 361–365.
Andreski, Stanislav. 1984. *Max Weber's Insights and Errors*. London: Routledge and Kegan Paul.
Angier, Natalie. 2008. "For Alien Life-Seekers, New Reason to Hope." *New York Times*, June 24, F1, F4.
Atoji, Yoshio. 1984. *Sociology at the Turn of the Century*. Tokyo: Dobunkan.
Ayala, Francisco J. 1995. "The Myth of Eve: Molecular Biology and Human Origins." *Science* 270 (December 22): 1930–1936.
Barrow, John D. 1988. *The World within the World*. New York: Oxford University Press.
———. 1991. *Theories of Everything*. New York: Fawcett Columbine.
Bash, Harry H. 1989/1998. "A Scatter of Sociologies: Vertical Drift and the Quest for Theoretical Integration in Sociology." In *The Living Legacy of Marx, Durkheim and Weber*, ed. Richard Altschuler, pp. 537–565. New York: Gordian Knot.
Beetham, David. 1985. *Max Weber and the Theory of Modern Politics*. Cambridge: Polity.
Bellah, Robert N. 1959. "Durkheim and History." *American Sociological Review*, vol. 24, no. 4 (August): 447–461.
———. 1973. "Introduction." In *Émile Durkheim on Morality and Society: Selected Writings*, pp. ix–lv. Chicago: University of Chicago Press.
Bendix, Reinhard. 1960. *Max Weber: An Intellectual Portrait*. Garden City, NY: Doubleday.
Benton, Michael J. 2003. *When Life Nearly Died*. London: Thames and Hudson.

Berger, Peter L., and Thomas Luckmann. 1967. *The Social Construction of Reality*. New York: Doubleday Anchor.

Besnard, Philippe. 2000. "The Fortunes of Dukheim's *Suicide*: Reception and Legacy." In *Durkheim's Suicide: A Century of Research and Debate*, ed. W.S.F. Pickering and Geoffrey Walford, pp. 97–125. London: Routledge.

Biello, David. 2007. "Culture Speeds Up Human Evolution." *Scientific American*, December 10.

Blakeslee, Sandra. 2001. "Science's Elusive Realm: Life's Little Mysteries." *New York Times*, April 24, F3.

Blau, Peter M. 1989. "Structures of Social Positions and Structures of Social Relations." In *Theory Building in Sociology: Assessing Theoretical Cumulation*, ed. Jonathan H. Turner, pp. 43–59. Newbury Park, CA: Sage.

Blumer, Herbert. 1946. "Collective Behavior." In *New Outline of the Principles of Sociology*, ed. Alfred McClung Lee. New York: Barnes and Noble.

Bologh, Roslyn Wallach. 1984. "Max Weber and the Dilemma of Rationality." In *Max Weber's Political Sociology*, ed. Ronald M. Glassman and Vatro Murvar, pp. 175–184. Westport, CT: Greenwood.

———. 1990. *Love or Greatness*. London: Unwin Hyman.

Bosse, Tibor, and Jan Treuer. 2006. "Formal Interpretation of a Multi-Agent Societry as a Single Agent." *Journal of Artificial Societies and Social Simulation*, vol. 9, no. 2 (March).

Bottomore, Tom. 1981. "A Marxist Consideration of Durkheim." *Social Forces*, vol. 59, no. 4 (June): 902–917.

Bottomore, Tom, and Robert Nisbet. 1978. "Structuralism." In *History of Sociological Analysis*, ed. Tom Bottomore and Robert Nisbet, pp. 557–599. New York: Basic Books.

Bradley, Raymond Trevor. 1987. *Charisma and Social Structure*. New York: Paragon.

Braithwaite, Richard Bevan. 1960. *Scientific Explanation*. New York: Harper.

Brodie, Bernard, and Fawn Brodie. 1962. *From Crossbow to H-Bomb*. New York: Dell.
Broom, Leonard. 1959. "Social Differentiation and Stratification." In *Sociology Today*, ed. Robert K. Merton, Leonard Broom, and Leonard S. Cottrell, Jr. New York: Basic Books.
Brubaker, Rogers. 1984. *The Limits of Rationality: an Essay on the Social and Moral Thought of Max Weber*. London: Allen and Unwin.
Buckley, Walter. 1967. *Sociology and Modern Systems Theory*. New York: Dryden.
Bueno de Mesquita, Bruce. 2002. *Predicting Politics*. Columbus: Ohio State University Press.
Burger, Thomas. 1977. "Max Weber, Interpretive Sociology, and the Sense of Historical Science: A Positivistic Conception of Verstehen," *Sociological Quarterly* 18 (Spring): 165–175.
———. 1985. "Power and Stratification: Max Weber and Beyond." In *Theory of Liberty, Legitimacy and Power*, ed. Vatro Murvar. Boston: Routledge and Kegan Paul.
———. 1987. *Max Weber's Theory of Concept Formation*. Expanded ed. Durham, NC: Duke University Press.
Burt, Ronald S. 1992. *Structural Holes: The Social Structure of Competition*. Cambridge: Harvard University Press.
Campbell, Donald T. 1958. "Common Fate, Similarity, and Other Indices of the Status of Aggregates of Persons as Social Entities." *Behavioural Sciences* 3:14–25.
———. 1965. "Variation and Selective Retention in Socio-Cultural Evolution." In *Social Change in Developing Areas*, ed. Herbert R. Barringer et al., pp. 19–49. Cambridge, MA: Schenkman.
Canup, Robin. 1999. "Big Bang, New Moon," http://www.swri.org/3pubs/ttoday/spring99/moon.htm.
Čapek, Karel. 1923. *R.U.R. (Rossum's Universal Robots): A Fantastic Melodrama*. Garden City, NY: Doubleday.
Clausewitz, Carl von. 1966. *On War*. London: Routledge and Kegan Paul.

Cohen, Joel E. 1995. *How Many People Can the Earth Support?* New York: Norton.
Coleman, James S. 1990. *Foundations of Social Theory.* Cambridge: Harvard University Press.
Collins, Randall. 1986. *Weberian Sociological Theory.* Cambridge: Cambridge University Press.
———. 1994. *Four Sociological Traditions.* New York: Oxford University Press.
Comte, Auguste. 1896. *The Positive Philosophy of Auguste Comte.* 3 vols. London: Bell.
———. 1975. *Auguste Comte and Positivism*, ed. Gertrud Lenzer. New York: Harper Torchbooks.
Contractor, Noshir S., and David R. Siebold. 1993. "Theoretical Frameworks for the Study of Structuring Processes in Group Decision Support Systems." *Human Communication Research*, vol. 19, no. 4 (June): 528–563.
Cooley, Charles Horton. 1956. *The Two Major Works of Charles H. Cooley: Social Organization, Human Nature and the Social Order.* Glencoe, IL: Free Press.
Cormack, Patricia. 1996. "The Paradox of Durkheim's Manifesto: Reconsidering "The Rules of Sociological Method." *Theory and Society*, vol. 25, issue 1 (February): 85–104.
Coser, Lewis A. 1977. *Masters of Sociological Thought.* New York: Harcourt Brace Jovanovich.
Cottrell, Fred. 1955. *Energy and Society.* New York: McGraw-Hill.
Craib, Ian. 1997. *Classical Social Theory.* New York: Oxford.
Cutright, Phillips, and Robert M. Fernquist. 2001. "The Relative Gender Gap in Suicide: Social Integration, the Culture of Suicide, and Period Effects in 20 Developed Countries, 1955–1994." *Social Science Research* 30:76–99.
Darwin, Charles. 1968. *The Origin of Species.* New York: Viking Penguin.
———. 1981. *The Descent of Man, and Selection in Relation to Sex.* Princeton: Princeton University Press.

Davidsson, Paul. 2002. "Agent Based Social Simulation: A Computer Science View." *Journal of Artificial Societies and Social Simulation*, vol. 5, no. 1. http://jasss.soc.surrey.ac.uk/5/1/7.html.

Dawkins, Richard. 1987. *The Blind Watchmaker*. New York: Norton.

Dawood, N. J. 1969. "Introduction." In Ibn Khaldûn, *The Muqaddimah: An Introduction to History* (abridged and edited), vii–xiv. Bollingen Series. Princeton: Princeton University Press.

Diamond, Jared. 1999. *Guns, Germs, and Steel*. New York: Norton.

Dohrenwend, Bruce P. 1990. "Egoism, Altruism, Anomie, and Fatalism: A Conceptual Analysis of Durkheim's Types." In *Émile Durkheim: Critical Assessments*, 3:22–33. London: Routledge.

Duong, Deborah Vakas, and John Grefenstette. 2005. "SISTER: A Symbolic Interactionist Simulation of Trade and Emergent Roles." *Journal of Artificial Societies and Social Simulation*, vol. 8, no. 1. http://jasss.soc.surrey.ac.uk/8/1/1.html.

Durkheim, Émile. 1960. "La sociologie et son domaine scientifique." In *Ou va la sociologie Francaise*? ed. Armand Cuvillier, pp. 177–208. Paris: Librairie Marcel Riviere.

———. 1986a. *De la division du travail social*. Paris: Quadrige/PUF.

———. 1912. *Le suicide*. Paris: Librairie Félix Alcan.

———. 1951. *Suicide*. New York: Free Press.

———. 1953. *Pragmatism and Sociology*. Cambridge: Cambridge University Press.

———. 1955. *Pragmatisme et Sociologie (cours inédit; prononcé a la Sorbonne en 1913–1914 et restitué par Armand Cuvillier d'après des notes d'étudiants)*. Paris: Librairie Philosophique J. Vrin.

———. 1956. *Education and Sociology*. Glencoe, IL: Free Press.

———. 1960a. "The Dualism of Human Nature and Its Social Conditions." In *Émile Durkheim, 1858–1917*, ed. Kurt H. Wolff, pp. 325–340. Columbus: Ohio State University Press.

———. 1960b. "Prefaces to L'Annee Sociologique." In *Émile Durkheim, 1858–1917*, ed. Kurt H. Wolff, pp. 341–353. Columbus: Ohio State University Press.

———. 1960c. "Sociology and Its Scientific Field." In *Émile Durkheim, 1858–1917*, ed. Kurt H. Wolff, pp. 354–375. Columbus: Ohio State University Press.

———. 1960d. "Sociology." In *Émile Durkheim, 1858–1917*, ed. Kurt H. Wolff, pp. 376–385. Columbus: Ohio State University Press.

———. 1960e. "Pragmatism and Sociology." In *Émile Durkheim, 1858–1917*, ed. Kurt H. Wolff, pp. 386–436. Columbus: Ohio State University Press.

———. 1968 (1912). *Les formes élémentaires de la vie religieuse*. Paris, France: Presses Universitaires de France.

———. 1973a. *On Morality and Society*. Chicago: University of Chicago.

———. 1973b. *Moral Education*. New York: Free Press.

———. 1974. *Sociology and Philosophy*. New York: Free Press.

———. 1978a. "Introduction to the Sociology of the Family." In *On Institutional Analysis*, pp. 205–228. Chicago: University of Chicago Press.

———. 1978b. "The Conjugal Family." In *On Institutional Analysis*, pp. 229–239. Chicago: University of Chicago Press.

———. 1978c. "Divorce by Mutual Consent." In *On Institutional Analysis*, pp. 240–252. Chicago: University of Chicago Press.

———. 1979. *Durkheim: Essays on Morals and Education*. London: Routledge and Kegan Paul.

———. 1981. "The Realm of Sociology as a Science." *Social Forces*, vol. 59, no. 4 (June): 1054–1070.

———. 1982a. "The Rules of Sociological Method." In *The Rules of Sociological Method and Selected Texts on Sociology and Its Method*, pp. 31–163. New York: Free Press.

———. 1982b. "Sociology and the Social Sciences." In *The Rules of Sociological Method and Selected Texts on Sociology and Its Method*, pp. 175–208. New York: Free Press.

———. 1982c. "Debate on the Relationship between Ethnology and Sociology." In *The Rules of Sociological Method and Selected Texts on Sociology and Its Method*, pp. 209–235. New York: Free Press.

———. 1982d. "Social Morphology." In *The Rules of Sociological Method and Selected Texts on Sociology and Its Method*, pp. 241–242. New York: Free Press.

———. 1982e. "The Method of Sociology." In *The Rules of Sociological Method and Selected Texts on Sociology and Its Method*, pp. 245–247. New York: Free Press.

———. 1983. *Durkheim and the Law*. New York: St. Martin's Press.

———. 1984. *The Division of Labor in Society*. New York: Free Press.

———. 1986b (1895). *Les règles de la méthode sociologique*. Paris, France: Quadrige/PUF.

———. 1986c. *Durkheim on Politics and the State*. Cambridge, UK: Polity.

———. 1992. *Professional Ethics and Civic Morals*. New York: Routledge.

———. 1994. *Durkheim on Religion*. Atlanta: Scholars Press.

———. 1995. *The Elementary Forms of Religious Life*. New York: Free Press.

Durkheim, Emile, and Marcel Mauss. 1963. *Primitive Classification*. Chicago: University of Chicago Press.

Dyer, Geoff. 2007. "Century's Playlist." *New York Times Book Review*, October 28, pp. 1, 9.

Eisenstadt, S. N. 1968. "Introduction." In *Max Weber on Charisma and Institution Building*, ed. S. N. Eisenstadt, pp. ix–lvi. Chicago: University of Chicago Press.

Emirbayer, Mustafa. 1996. "Useful Durkheim." *Sociological Theory*, vol. 3 (July): 109–130.

Engels, Frederick. 1969. "The Origin of the Family, Private Property and the State." In *Karl Marx and Frederick Engels, Selected Works*, 3: 204–334. Moscow: Progress.

Epstein, Joshua M., and Robert Axtell. 1996. *Growing Artificial Societies: Social Science from the Bottom Up*. Washington, DC: Brookings Institution Press.

Erickson, Kai. 1966. *Wayward Puritans*. New York: Wiley.

———. 1986. "On Work and Alienation." *American Sociological Review*, vol. 51 (February): 1–8.

Espinas, Alfred Victor. 1977. *Des sociétés animales*. New York: Arno.
Fagan, Brian. 2008. *The Great Warming*. New York: Bloomsbury.
Fanon, Frantz. 1968. *The Wretched of the Earth*. New York: Grove.
Fararo, Thomas J., and John Skvoretz. 2002. "Theoretical Integration and Generative Structuralism." In *New Directions in Contemporary Sociological Theory*, ed. Joseph Berger and Morris Zelditch, Jr., pp. 295–316. New York: Rowman and Littlefield.
Feigl, Herbert. 1953. "Notes on Causality." In *Readings in the Philosophy of Science*, ed. Herbert Feigl and May Brodbeck, pp. 408–418. New York: Appleton-Century-Crofts.
Fenton, Steve, with Robert Reiner and Ian Hamnett. 1984. *Durkheim and Modern Sociology*. New York: Cambridge University Press.
Ferguson, R. Brian. 2006. "Archaeology, Cultural Anthropology, and the Origins and Intensifications of War." In *The Archaeology of Warfare: Prehistories of Raiding and Conquest*, ed. Elizabeth N. Arkush and Marx W. Allen, pp. 469–523. Gainesville: University Press of Florida.
Feynman, Richard P. 1985. *QED: The Strange Theory of Light and Matter*. Princeton: Princeton University Press.
Fields, Karen E. 1995. "Translator's Introduction." In Émile Durkheim, *The Elementary Forms of Religious Life*, pp. xvii–lxxiii. New York: Free Press.
———. 1996. "Durkheim and the Idea of Soul," *Theory and Society* 25:193–203.
Flack, Jessica. 2007. "Complex Form Evolving." *SFI Bulletin*, vol. 22, no. 1:52–57.
Freud, Sigmund. 1959. *Group Psychology and the Analysis of the Ego*. New York: Norton.
———. 1962. *Civilization and Its Discontents*. New York: Norton.
Gane, Mike. 2000. "The Deconstruction of Social Action: The 'Reversal' of Durkheimian Methodology from *The Rules* to *Suicide*." In *Durkheim's* Suicide*: A Century of Research and Debate*, ed. W.S.F. Pickering and Geoffrey Walford, pp. 22–35. London: Routledge.

———. 2001. "Durkheim's Project for a Sociological Science." In *Handbook of Social Theory*, ed. George Ritzer and Barry Smart, pp. 79–88. Thousand Oaks, CA: Sage.

Gerstein, Dean. 1983. "Durkheim's Paradigm: Reconstructing a Social Theory," *Sociological Theory* 1:234–25.

Gerth, H. H., and C. Wright Mills. 1946. "Introduction." In *Essays from Max Weber*, ed. H. H. Gerth and C. Wright Mills, pp. 3–75. New York: Oxford.

Giddens, Anthony. 1979. *Émile Durkheim*. New York: Penguin.

Giddings, Franklin Henry. 1896. *The Principles of Sociology*. New York: Macmillan.

Gilbert, Margaret. 1994. "Durkheim and Social Facts." In *Debating Durkheim*, ed. W.S.F. Pickering and H. Martins, pp. 86–109. London: Routledge.

Goldspink, Chris. 2000. "Modelling Social Systems as Complex: Towards a Social Simulation Meta-Model," *Journal of Artificial Societies and Social Simulation*, vol. 3, no. 2. http://jasss.soc.surrey.ac.uk/3/2/1.html.

———. 2002. "Methodological Implications of Complex System Approaches to Sociality: Simulation as a Foundation for Knowledge." *Journal of Artificial Societies and Social Simulation*, vol. 5, no. 1. http://jasss.soc.surrey.ac.uk/5/1/3.html.

Goleman, Daniel. 1991. "Happy or Sad, a Mood Can Prove Contagious." *New York Times*, October 15, C1, C8.

Goldstone, Jack A. 2002. "Theory Development in the Study of Revolutions." In *New Directions in Contemporary Sociological Theory*, ed. Joseph Berger and Morris Zelditch, Jr. , pp. 194–226. New York: Rowman and Littlefield.

Goody, Jack, and I. Watt. 1972. "The Consequences of Literacy." In *Language and Social Context*, ed. Pier Paolo Giglioli. Baltimore: Penguin.

Gouldner, Alvin W. 1976. *The Dialectic of Ideology and Technology*. New York: Seabury.

Greene, Brian. 2004. *The Fabric of the Cosmos*. New York: Knopf.

Gribbin, John. 1995. *Schrödinger's Kittens*. London: Weidenfeld and Nicolson.
Griffith, Samuel B. 1963. "Preface." In Sun Tzu, *The Art of War*, pp. ix–xi. New York: Oxford University Press.
Habermas, Jurgen. 1971. *Knowledge and Human Interests*. Boston: Beacon Press.
Heckathorn, Douglas D. 2002. "Development of a Theory of Collective Action: From the Emergence of Norms to AIDS Prevention and the Analysis of Social Structure." In *New Directions in Contemporary Sociological Theory*, ed. Joseph Berger and Morris Zelditch, Jr., pp. 79–108. New York: Rowman and Littlefield.
Heider, Fritz. 1958. *The Psychology of Interpersonal Relations*. New York: Wiley.
Hempel, Carl G. 1965. *Aspects of Scientific Explanation*. New York: Free Press.
Hennis, Wilhelm. 1983. "Max Weber's 'Central Question.'" *Economy and Society* vol. 12, no. 2:135–180.
Hindess, Barry. 1987. "Rationality and the Characterization of Modern Society." In *Max Weber, Rationality and Modernity*, ed. Sam Whimster and Scott Lash, pp. 137<en>53. London: Allen and Unwin.
Hinkle, Roscoe C., Jr. 1960. "Durkheim in American Sociology." In *Émile Durkheim, 1858–1917*, ed. Kurt H. Wolff, pp. 267–295. Columbus: Ohio State University Press.
Hogan, James P. 1979. *The Two Faces of Tomorrow*. New York: Ballantine.
Holland, John H. 1998. *Emergence: From Chaos to Order*. Cambridge, MA: Perseus.
Hölldobler, Bert, and Edward O. Wilson. 1990. *The Ants*. Cambridge: Harvard University Press.
Huff, Toby E. 1984. *Max Weber and the Methodology of the Social Sciences*. New Brunswick, NJ: Transaction Books.

Huitt, William G., and Sheila C. Cain. 2005. "An Overview of the Conative Domain." In *Educational Psychology Interactive*, pp. 1–20. Valdosta, GA.: Valdosta State University.

Hunt, Lynn. 1988. "The Sacred and the French Revolution." In *Durkheimian Sociology: Cultural Studies*, ed. Jeffrey C. Alexander, pp. 25–43. New York: Cambridge University Press.

Ibn Khaldûn. 1958. *The Muqaddimah: An Introduction to History*, vol. 2, 2nd ed. Bollingen Series 43. Princeton: Princeton University Press.

———. 1967. *The Muqaddimah: An Introduction to History*, vol. 1, 2nd ed., with corrections and augmented bibliography. Bollingen Series 43. Princeton: Princeton University Press.

———. 1969. *The Muqaddimah: An Introduction to History*, abridged and edited. Bollingen Series. Princeton: Princeton University Press.

Inbar, Michael. 1979. *The Future of Bureaucracy*. Beverly Hills: Sage.

Jastrow, Robert. 1981. *The Enchanted Loom*. New York: Simon and Schuster.

Jepperson, Ronald L. 2002. "The Development and Application of Sociological Neoinstitutionalism." In *New Directions in Contemporary Sociological Theory*, ed. Joseph Berger and Morris Zelditch, Jr., pp. 229–266. New York: Rowman and Littlefield.

Jewell, Peter A. 1983. "Species Diversity and Environmental Carrying Capacity amongst Large Mammals and the Shift of Equilibria by Man." In *Malthus Past and Present,* ed. Dupaquier, Fauve-Chamoux, and Grebenik, pp. 365–377. New York: Academic Press.

Johnson, Barclay D. 1990. "Durkheim's One Cause of Suicide." In *Émile Durkheim: Critical Assessments*, ed. Peter Hamilton, 3:34–51. London: Routledge.

Jones, Robert Alun. 1986. *Émile Durkheim: An Introduction to Four Major Works*. Beverley Hills: Sage.

———. 1998. "Religion and Science in *The Elementary Forms*." In *On Durkheim's Elementary Forms of Religious Life*, ed. N. J. Allen,

W.S.F. Pickering, and W. Watts Miller, pp. 39–52. London: Routledge.

———. 1999. *The Development of Durkheim's Social Realism*. New York: Cambridge University Press.

Jones, Susan Stedman. 2001. *Durkheim Reconsidered*. Cambridge: Polity.

Kalberg, Stephen. 1980. "Max Weber's Types of Rationality: Cornerstones for the Analysis of Rationalization Processes in History." *American Journal of Sociology*, vol. 85, no. 5 (March): 1145–1179.

———. 2002. "Introduction to *The Protestant Ethic*." In Max Weber, *The Protestant Ethic and The Spirit of Capitalism*, pp. xi–lxxvi, 3rd Roxbury ed. Los Angeles: Roxbury.

Kanter, James. 2008. "One in 4 Mammals Threatened with Extinction, Group Finds." *New York Times*, October 7, A14.

Kauffman, Stuart. 1995. *At Home in the Universe*. New York: Oxford University Press.

———. 2000. *Investigations*. New York: Oxford University Press.

Kaufman-Osborn, Timothy V. 1988. "Modernity's Myth of Facts." *Theory and Society* 17:121–147.

Kellner, Douglas. 1985. "Critical Theory, Max Weber, and the Dialectics of Domination." In *A Marx-Weber Dialogue*, ed. Robert J. Antonio and Ronald M. Glassman, pp. 89–116. Lawrence: University Press of Kansas.

Keynes, Richard. 1983. "Malthus and Biological Equilibria." In *Malthus Past and Present*, ed. Dupaquier, Fauve-Chamoux, and Grebenik, pp. 359–364. New York: Academic Press.

Klein, Richard G. 1989. *The Human Career*, 2nd ed. Chicago: University of Chicago Press.

Knobe, Joshua, Ken D. Olum, and Alexander Vilenkin. 2006. "Philosophical Implications of Inflationary Cosmology." *British Journal for the Philosophy of Science*, vol. 57, no. 1:47–67.

Kroeber, A. L., and Talcott Parsons. 1958. "The Concepts of Culture and of Social System." *American Sociological Review*, vol. 23 (October): 582–583.

Kuper, Leo. 1969. "Plural Societies: Perspectives and Problems." In *Pluralism in Africa*, ed. Leo Kuper and M. G. Smith. Berkeley: University of California Press.

Lawrence, Bruce B. 2005. "Introduction to the 2005 Edition." In *The Muqaddimah: An Introduction to History*, pp. vii–xxv. Princeton: Princeton University Press.

Leakey, Richard, and Roger Lewin. 1992. *Origins Reconsidered*. New York: Doubleday.

LeBon, Gustave. 1960. *The Crowd*. New York: Viking.

Lenski, Gerhard E. 1975. "Social Structure in Evolutionary Perspective." In *Approaches to the Study of Social Structure*, ed. Peter M. Blau. New York: Free Press.

Levine, Donald N. 1981. "Rationality and Freedom: Weber and Beyond." *Sociological Inquiry*, vol. 51, no. 1:5–25.

Levi-Setti, Riccardo. 1993. *Trilobites*. Chicago: University of Chicago Press.

Levy, Marion J., Jr. 1972. *Modernization: Latecomers and Survivors*. New York: Basic Books.

Lim, May, Richard Metzler, and Yaneer Bar-Yam. 2007. "Global Pattern Formation and Ethnic/Cultural Violence." *Science*, vol. 317 (September 14): 1540–1544.

Lindholm, Charles. 1990. *Charisma*. Cambridge: Basil Blackwell.

Lindley, David. 2007. *Uncertainty: Einstein, Heisenberg, Bohr, and the Struggle for the Soul of Science*. New York: Doubleday.

Lorenz, Konrad. 1970. *Studies in Animal and Human Behaviour*. 2 vols. Cambridge: Harvard University Press.

Lukes, Steven. 1975. *Émile Durkheim: His Life and Work*. New York: Peregrine Books.

———. 1979. "Some Problems about Rationality." In *Rationality*, ed. Bryan R. Wilson, pp. 194–213. Oxford: Basil Blackwell.

———. 1982. "Introduction." In Émile Durkheim, *The Rules of Sociological Method and Selected Texts on Sociology and Its Method*, pp. 1–27. New York: Free Press.

———. 1990 (1971). "Prolegomena to the Interpretation of Durkheim." In *Émile Durkheim: Critical Assessments*, ed. Peter Hamilton, 2:318–342. London: Routledge.

Lyman, Sanford. 1984. "The Science of History and the Theory of Social Change." In *Max Weber's Political Sociology*, ed. Ronald M. Glassman and Vatro Murvar, pp. 189–199. Westport, CT: Greenwood.

Macy, Michael W., and Robert Willer. 2002. "From Factors to Actors: Computational Sociology and Agent-Based Modeling." *Annual Review of Sociology* 28:143–166.

Malthus, Thomas Robert. 1966. *First Essay on Population*. New York: Macmillan.

Mannheim, Karl. 1955. *Ideology and Utopia*. New York: Harvest Books.

Marcuse, Herbert. 1971. "Industrialization and Capitalism." In *Max Weber and Sociology Today*, ed. Otto Stammer, pp. 133–151. New York: Harper and Row.

Marks, Stephen R. 1974. "Durkheim's Theory of Anomie." *American Journal of Sociology*, vol. 80, no. 2: 329–363.

Martindale, Don, and Johannes Riedel. 1958. "Max Weber's Sociology of Music." In Max Weber, *The Rational and Social Foundations of Music*. Carbondale: Southern Illinois University Press.

Marx, Karl. 1922. *Das Kapital*. Hamburg, Germany: Meissner.

———. 1964. *Economic and Philosophic Manuscripts of 1844*. New York: International.

———. 1967. *Capital*, 3 vols., unabridged. New York: International.

———. 1973. *Grundrisse*. New York: Vintage.

Marx, Karl, and Friedrich Engels. 1969. *Selected Works*, 3 vols. Moscow: Progress.

Mead, George Herbert. 1962. *Mind, Self, and Society*. Chicago: University of Chicago Press.

Merton, Robert K. 1934 (1998). "Durkheim's *Division of Labor in Society*." Reprinted in *The Living Legacy of Marx, Durkheim and Weber*, ed. Richard Altschuler, pp. 372–381. New York: Gordian Knot.

———. 1957. *Social Theory and Social Structure*, rev. and enl. ed. Glencoe, IL: Free Press.

———. 1973. *The Sociology of Science*. Chicago: University of Chicago Press.

Miller, George A., Eugene Galanter, and Karl H. Pribam. 1960. *Plans and the Structure of Behavior*. New York: Holt, Rinehart and Winston.

Mommsen, Wolfgang J. 1974. *The Age of Bureaucracy: Perspectives on the Political Sociology of Max Weber*. Oxford: Basil Blackwell.

Moody, James, Daniel McFarland, and Skye Bender-deMoll. 2005. "Dynamic Network Visualization." *American Journal of Sociology*, vol. 110, no. 4 (January): 1206–1241.

Morowitz, Harold J. 2002. *The Emergence of Everything: How the World BecameComplex*. New York: Oxford University Press.

Moss, Scott, and Bruce Edmonds. 2005. "Sociology and Simulation: Statistical and Qualitative Cross-Validation." *American Journal of Sociology*, vol. 110, no. 4 (January): 1095–1131.

Naegele, Kaspar D. 1958. "Attachment and Alienation: Complementary Aspects of the Work of Durkheim and Simmel." *American Journal of Sociology*, vol. 63, no. 6 (May): 580–589.

Nisbet, Robert A. 1965. "Émile Durkheim." In *Émile Durkheim*, ed. Robert A. Nisbet, pp. 9–102. Englewood Cliffs NJ: Prentice-Hall.

Nozick, Robert. 1993. *The Nature of Rationality*. Princeton: Princeton University Press.

Ogburn, William Fielding. 1933. *Social Change*. New York: Viking.

Ong, Walter J. 1971. *Rhetoric, Romance, and Technology*. Ithaca: Cornell University Press.

Oliver, Pamela E., and Gerald Marwell. 2002. "Recent Developments in Critical Mass Theory." In *New Directions in Contemporary Sociological Theory*, ed. Joseph Berger and Morris Zeldith, Jr., pp. 172–193. New York: Rowman and Littlefield.

Orum, Anthony M. 1988. "Political Sociology." In *Handbook of Sociology*, ed. Neil J. Smelser. Berkeley: Sage.

Pareto, Vilfredo. 1935. *The Mind and Society.* 4 vols. New York: Harcourt Brace.
Parkin, Frank. 1982. *Max Weber.* Chichester, UK: Ellis Horwood.
Parsons, Talcott. 1937. *The Structure of Social Action.* Glencoe, IL.: Free Press.
———. 1949. *The Structure of Social Action.* Glencoe, IL: Free Press.
———. 1960. Durkheim's Contribution to the Theory of Integration of Social Systems." In *Émile Durkheim, 1858–1917*, ed. Kurt H. Wolff, pp. 118–153. Columbus: Ohio State University Press.
———. 1961. "An Outline of the Social System." In *Theories of Society: Foundations of Modern Sociological Theory*, ed. Talcott Parsons et al, pp. 30–79. New York: Free Press.
Parsons, Talcott, and Edward A. Shils. 1951. "Categories of the Orientation and Organization of Action." In *Toward a General Theory of Action*, ed. Talcott Parsons and Edward A. Shils, pp. 53–109. New York: Harper.
Partridge, Eric. 1959. *Origins.* New York: Macmillan.
Pascal, R. 1947. "Introduction." In *The German Ideology (Parts I and III)*, pp. ix–xviii. New York: International.
Pattee, Howard H., ed. 1973. *Hierarchy Theory: The Challenge of Complex Systems.* New York: Braziller.
Peyre, Henri. 1960. "Durkheim: The Man, His Time, and His Intellectual Background." In *Émile Durkheim, 1858–1917*, ed. Kurt H. Wolff, pp. 3–31. Columbus: Ohio State University Press.
Pickering, W.S.F. 2000. "Reading the Conclusion." In *Durkheim's Suicide: A Century of Research and Debate*, ed. W.S.F. Pickering and Geoffrey Walford, pp. 66–80. London: Routledge.
Pope, Whitney. 1976. *Durkheim's Suicide: A Classic Analyzed.* Chicago: University of Chicago Press.
Popper, Karl R. 1961. *The Logic of Scientific Discovery.* New York: Science Editions.
Rawls, Anne Warfield. 1996. "Durkheim's Epistemology: The Neglected Argument." *American Journal of Sociology*, vol. 102, no. 2 (September): 430–482.

Reed, John. 1960. *Ten Days That Shook the World.* New York: Modern Library.
Ritzer, George. 1992. *Metatheorizing in Sociology.* Lexington, MA: Lexington.
Ritzer, George, and Richard Bell. 1981. "Émile Durkheim: Exemplar for an Integrated Sociological Paradigm?" *Social Forces*, vol. 59, no. 4 (June): 966–995.
Robertson, Roland. 1990. "Mapping the Global Condition: Globalization as the Central Concept." *Theory, Culture and Society* 7 (June): 15–30.
Sample, Ian. 2006. "Earth Facing 'Catastrophic' Loss of Species." *Guardian* (July 20).
Sayer, Derek. 1991. *Capitalism and Modernity: An Excursus on Mark and Weber.* London: Routledge.
Schluchter, Wolfgang. 1979. "The Paradox of Rationalization: On the Relation of Ethics and World." In *Max Weber's Vision of History*, ed. Guenther Roth and Wolfgang Schluchter, pp. 11–64. Berkeley: University of California Press.
———. 1989. *Rationalism, Religion, and Domination: A Weberian Perspective.* Berkeley: University of California Press.
Schroeder, Ralph. 1992. *Max Weber and the Sociology of Culture.* Hawthorne, NY: Aldine.
Scully, Matthew. 2006. "God Is Green." *New York Times Book Review*, September 10, p. 9.
Segady, Thomas W. 1987. *Value, Neo-Kantianism and the Development of Weberian Methodology.* New York: Peter Lang.
Semple, Ellen Churchill. 1933. *American History and Its Geographic Conditions.* Boston: Houghton Mifflin.
Shibutani, Tamotsu. 1968. "A Cybernetic Approach to Motivation." In *Modern Systems Research for the Behavioral Scientist*, ed. Walter Buckley, pp. 330–336. Chicago: Aldine.
Shils, Edward. 1987. "Max Weber and the World since 1920." In *Max Weber and His Contemporaries*, ed. Wolfgang J. Mommsen and Jurgen Osterhammel, pp. 547–573. London: Allen and Unwin.
Shubin, Neil. 2008. *Your Inner Fish.* New York. Pantheon.

Sica, Alan. 1988. *Weber, Irrationality, and Social Order.* Berkeley: University of California Press.
Simmel, Georg. 1950. *The Sociology of Georg Simmel.* Glencoe, IL: Free Press.
———. 1955. *Conflict and the Web of Group Affiliations.* New York: Free Press.
Simon, Herbert A. 1965. "Causal Ordering and Identifiability." In *Cause and Effect*, ed. Daniel Lerner, pp. 157–189. New York: Free Press.
———. 1973. "The Organization of Complex Systems." In *Hierarchy Theory: The Challenge of Complex Systems*, ed. Howard H. Pattee, pp. 1–28. New York: George Braziller.
Smith, Adam. 1937. *An Inquiry into the Nature and Causes of the Wealth of Nations.* New York: Modern Library.
Sowell, Thomas. 1996. *Migrations and Cultures.* New York: Basic Books.
Spencer, Herbert. 1898. *The Principles of Sociology.* 3 vols. New York: Appleton.
———. 1961. *The Study of Sociology.* Ann Arbor: University of Michigan Press.
Stoeckle, Mary Y., and Paul D. N. Hebert. 2008. "Barcode of Life." *Scientific American*, vol. 299, no. 4 (October): 82–86.
Sun Tzu. 1963. *The Art of War.* New York: Oxford University Press.
Swatos, William H., Jr. 1984. "Revolution and Charisma in a Rationalized World: Weber Revisited and Extended." In *Max Weber's Political Sociology*, ed. Ronald M. Glassman and Matro Murvar, pp. 201–215. Westport, CT: Greenwood.
Swidler, Ann. 1973. "The Concept of Rationality in the Work of Max Weber." *Sociological Inquiry*, vol. 43, no. 1:35–42.
Tekla, Tendzin N., and Whitney Pope. 1985. "The Force Imagery in Durkheim: The Integration of Theory, Metatheory, and Method." *Sociological Theory*, vol. 3, number 1 (Spring): 74–88.
Tenbruck, Friedrich H. 1980. "The Problem of Thematic Unity in the Works of Max Weber." *British Journal of Sociology* 31 (September): 316<en>51.

TenHouten, Warren. 1998. "Dual Symbolic Classification and the Primary Emotions." In *The Living Legacy of Marx, Durkheim and Weber*, ed. Richard Altschuler, pp. 409–434. New York: Gordian Knot.

Thomas, William I. and Dorothy Swaine. 1928. *The Child in America*. New York: Knopf.

Thompson, Kenneth. 1998. "Durkheim and Sacred Identity." In *On Durkheim's Elementary Forms of Religious Life*, ed. N. J. Allen, W.S.F. Pickering, and W. Watts Miller pp. 92–104. London: Routledge.

Tilly, Charles. 1981. *As Sociology Meets History*, New York: Academic.

Tiryakian, Edward A. 1962. *Sociologism and Existentialism*. Englewood Cliffs, NJ: Prentice-Hall.

———. 1978. "Émile Durkheim." In *A History of Sociological Analysis*, ed. Tom Bottomore and Robert Nisbet, pp. 187–236. New York: Basic Books.

Tominaga, Ken'ichi. 1989. "Max Weber and the Modernization of China and Japan." In *Cross-National Research in Sociology*, ed. Melvin L. Kohn, 125–146. London: Sage.

Traugott, Mark. 1978. "A Note on the Translations." In Émile Durkheim, *On Institutional Analysis*, pp. ix–xii. Chicago: University of Chicago Press.

———. 1978b. "Introduction." In Émile Durkheim, *On Institutional Analysis*, pp. 1–39. Chicago: University of Chicago Press.

Turner, Bryan S. 1992. "Preface to the Second Edition." In Émile Durkheim, *Professional Ethics and Civic Morals*, pp. xiii–xlii. New York: Routledge.

Turner, Jonathan H., Leonard Beeghley, and Charles H. Powers. 2002. *The Emergence of Sociological Theory*, 5th ed. Belmont, CA: Wadsworth Thomson Learning.

Van Fraassen, Bas C. 1991. *Quantum Mechanics: An Empiricist View*. New York: Oxford University Press.

Veblen, Thorstein. 1979. *The Theory of the Leisure Class*. New York: Penguin.

Vilenkin, Alex. 2006. *Many Worlds in One*. New York: Hill and Wang.

Voight, Benjamin F., Sridhar Kudaravalli, Xiaoquon Wen, and Jonathan K. Pritchard. 2006. "A Map of Recent Positive Selection in the Human Genome." *PLoS Biology*, vol. 4, no. 3 (March): 72.
Von Bertalanffy, Ludwig. 1956. "General System Theory." *General Systems Yearbook*, 1:1–10.
Wagner, David G., and Joseph Berger. 2002. "Expectation States Theory: An Evolving Research Program." In *New Directions in Contemporary Sociological Theory*, ed. Joseph Berger and Morris Zelditch, Jr., pp. 41–76. New York: Rowman and Littlefield.
Waldrop. M. Mitchell. 1992. *Complexity*. New York: Simon and Schuster.
Wallace, Walter L. 1983. *Principles of Scientific Sociology*. New York: Aldine.
———. 1994. *A Weberian Theory of Human Society: Structure and Evolution*. New Brunswick, NJ: Rutgers University Press.
——— 1997. *The Future of Ethnicity, Race, and Nationality*. Westport CT: Praeger.
Wallerstein, Immanuel. 1979. *The Capitalist World-Economy*. New York: Cambridge University Press.
Ward, Peter D., and Donald Brownlee. 2000. *Rare Earth*. New York: Copernicus, Springer-Verlag.
Weber, Max. 1946. *From Max Weber: Essays in Sociology*, ed. H. H.Gerth and C. Wright Mills. New York: Oxford University Press.
———. 1947. "Die Protestantische Ethik and der Geist des Kapitalismus." In *Gesammelte Aufsätze zur Religionssoziologie*, pp. 17–206. Tubingen: J.C.B. Mohr.
———. 1949. *The Methodology of the Social Sciences*. Glencoe, IL: Free Press.
——— 1958. *The Protestant Ethic and the Spirit of Capitalism*. New York: Scribners.
——— 1978. *Economy and Society*, 2 vols. Berkeley: University of California Press.

Weiss, Johannes. 1985. "On the Marxist Reception and Critique of Max Weber in Eastern Europe." In *A Marx-Weber Dialogue*, ed. Robert J. Antonio and Ronald M. Glassman. Lawrence: University Press of Kansas.

Wheeler, John Archibald. 1998. *Geons, Black Holes, and Quantum Foam*. New York: Norton.

White, Leslie. 1949. *The Science of Culture*. New York: Grove.

Wiley, Norbert. 1987. "Introduction." In *The Marx-Weber Debate*, ed. Norbert Wiley, pp. 7–27. Newbury Park, CA: Sage.

Willer, David, Henry A. Walker, Barry Markovsky, Robb Willer, Michael Lovaglia, Shane Thye, and Brent Simpson. 2002. "Network Exchange Theory." In *New Directions in Contemporary Sociological Theory*, ed. Joseph Berger and Morris Zelditch, Jr., pp. 109–144. New York: Rowman and Littlefield.

Wilson, Bryan R. 1979. "A Sociologist's Introduction." In *Rationality*, ed. Bryan R. Wilson, pp. vii–xviii. Oxford: Basil Blackwell.

Wilson, Edward O. 1975. *Sociobiology*. Cambridge: Harvard University Press.

Wrong, Dennis. 1970. "Introduction." In *Max Weber*. Englewood Cliffs, NJ: Prentice-Hall.

Wuthnow, Robert. 1987. *Meaning and Moral Order*. Berkeley: University of California Press.

———. 1988. "Sociology of Religion." In *Handbook of Sociology*, ed. Neil J. Smelser, pp. 473–509. Newbury Park, CA: Sage.

Zinsser, Hans. 1967. *Rats, Lice, and History*. New York: Bantam.

## More Detailed Table of Contents

**Introduction**
Human species extinction     3
Human species survival
    via evolution of individual anatomy and physiology     2
    via evolution of collective sociocultural phenomena     9
Sociocultural phenomena, defined generically     14
Societies, defined generically, 14
Societies, human, defined, 15
    Types of institutions constitutive of human societies     17
    Types of organizations constitutive of the human
       societal participant-organizing institution     17

**Malthus's and Darwin's Precursor Theories**
Malthus' positive checks and preventive checks on
    population as mechanisms of human societal survival     20
Darwin's competition, migration, and adaptive speciation
    of population as mechanisms of all terrestrial life's
    self-maintenance     22

**Durkheim's Core Theory**
Sociocultural self-maintenance     26
Role of the individual in human sociocultural self-maintenance     27
*The Division of Labor in Society* (social structure: segmental
    and organized; culture structure: mechanical and organic)     29
    Abnormalities in social structure     35
*Suicide* (social structure "integration" and culture structure
    "regulation")     41
    Abnormalities in social structure and culture structure     42
*Elementary Forms of Religious Life* (past origin of morality
    culture structure)     46
*Moral Education* (future source of moral culture structure)     58
Implicit long-term human species survival forecast     63

## Marx's Supplementary Theory

| | |
|---|---:|
| Marx's initial premises versus Durkheim's initial premises | 69 |
| Economic organizations: primary means of human societal and species survival | 70 |
| Thumbnail sketch of Marx's theory | 71 |
| Human labor-power and nonhuman instruments of labor | 72 |
|     Robots as the ultimate nonhuman instruments of labor | 77 |
|     Labor-process and modes of production | 80 |
|     Two meanings of "capital" | 81 |
|     Employer-employee economic division of labor | 83 |
|     Employee economic-political organizational revolution | 87 |
| Employer past contributions to human species survival | 88 |
| One implicit long-term human species survival forecast | 95 |

## Weber's Supplementary Theory

| | |
|---|---:|
| Conscious and unconscious human psychical behavior | 97 |
| Generic definition of rational psychical behavior | 99 |
|     Ten types of Weberian rationality | 102 |
|     Choosing among alternative means or among alternative ends | 111 |
| Ethical standards of behavior | 112 |
| Two types of Weberian nonrationality | 115 |
|     Charisma variably combines both types | 118 |
|     Some possible objects of charisma | 120 |
|     Durkheim's "sacred" versus Weber's "charisma" | 125 |
|     Unpredictability of charisma | 126 |
| Human physical behavior | 127 |
| *The Protestant Ethic and the Spirit of Capitalism* | 129 |
|     Routinization of human and nonhuman charismatic objects | 130 |
| Two opposing long-range human species survival forecasts | 135 |

## Ibn Khaldûn's, and Others,' Supplementary Theories

| | |
|---|---:|
| Social structure and culture structure | 138 |
| Culture structure "group feeling" | 139 |
| Physical force and violence | 140 |

Rise and fall of dynasties: oscillation of culture structures
of appetite and forgetfulness                                   141
Geography and technology in human sociocultural
phenomena                                                       144
Ibn Khaldûn's theoretical descendants on geography              147
Ibn Khaldûn's theoretical descendants on technology             149
Military and police political technology                        153
Technological defenses against cosmic threats                   157
Our own long-term human species survival forecasts              157

**Summary and Conclusion**
Geography and technology versus moral culture structure         164
Human competitiveness and class struggle                        167
Causal determinism and causal probabilism                       170
Concluding short-term species survival proposal                 176

**Appendix**
Durkheim's core human sociocultural self-maintenance theory     177
Durkheim's inconsistencies                                      182
Social structure and culture structure in Durkheim's theory     184

# Name Index

Albrow, Martin, 108, 208
Alexander, Jeffrey C., 178, 183
Alpert, Harry, 177
Andreski, Stanislav, 208, 209
Angier, Natalie, 157, 188
Atoji, Yoshio, 209
Axtell, Robert, 9, 12
Ayala, Francisco J., 188

Barrow, John D., 216, 217
Bar-Yam, Yaneer, 188
Beetham, David, 135, 208
Bell, Richard, 184, 188, 193
Bellah, Robert N., 52, 182, 184, 197, 214
Bendix, Reinhard, 208
Benton, Michael J., 187
Berger, Joseph, 216
Berger, Peter L., 49, 177
Besnard, Phillippe, 191, 197
Blakeslee, Sandra, 216
Blau, Peter, 181
Blumer, Herbert, 200
Bologh, Roslyn Wallach, 112, 207, 208
Bosse, Tibor, 188
Bottomore, Tom, 185
Bradley, Raymond Trevor, 124, 210
Braithwaite, Richard Bevan, 174
Brodie, Bernard, 154–156
Brodie, Fawn, 154–156
Brownlee, Donald, 5, 7, 23, 145, 168, 218
Brubaker, Rogers, 208
Buckley, Walter, 174
Bueno de Mesquita, Bruce, 182, 216

Burger, Thomas, 208
Burt, Ronald, 188

Calvin, John, 131, 132, 134, 211
Campbell, Donald T., 5, 8
Canup, Robin, 218
Čapek, Karel, 77
Chomsky, Noam, 217
Clarke, Arthur, 188
Cohen, Joel E., 23, 189, 190
Collins, Randall, 50, 180, 186, 197, 208, 215
Comte, Auguste, 25, 26, 170, 173, 199, 201, 211
Contractor, Noshir, 10
Cooley, Charles Horton, 36
Cormack, Patricia, 179, 182, 185, 191
Coser, Lewis A., 1
Cottrell, Fred, 150
Craib, Ian, 1
Cutright, Phillips, 197, 215

Darwin, Charles, 3, 4, 6, 7, 9, 11, 18, 21–24, 30, 31, 35, 72, 84, 90, 127, 144, 157, 162, 163, 168, 169, 188, 190, 201, 205, 216
Davidsson, Paul, 10
Dawkins, Richard, 22, 206, 216, 217
Dawood, N. J., 212
Diamond, Jared, 22, 148, 218
Dohrenwend, Bruce P., 197
Duncan, Otis Dudley, 179
Duong, Deborah Vakas, 188
Durkheim, Emile, 4, 11, 12, 14, 18, 23, 25–46, 48–65, 69,

70, 84, 91, 96, 117, 120,
123, 125–127, 133, 134,
137-139, 144, 150, 161–166,
168, 171–173, 177–189,
191–201, 206, 210, 213–215

Edmonds, Bruce, 188
Einstein, Albert, 1, 127, 215
Eisenstadt, S. N., 124
Emirbayer, Mustafa, 178, 188
Engels, Frederick, 11, 71, 72, 94,
150, 201, 202, 204
Epstein, Joshua M., 9, 12
Erikson, Kai T., 152
Espinas, Alfred Victor, 28

Fagan, Brian, 149
Fararo, Thomas J., 216
Feigl, Herbert, 215
Fenton, Steve, 181, 185
Ferguson, R. Brian, 153, 154
Fernquist, Robert M., 197, 215
Feynman, Richard P., 216
Fields, Karen E., 54, 183
Flack, Jessica, 195
Freud, Sigmund, 97, 120, 207,
213

Gane, Mike, 172, 178, 181, 197
Gerstein, Dean, 180
Gerth, H. H., 125
Giddens, Anthony, 36, 112, 182,
184, 208
Giddings, Franklin Henry, 36
Gilbert, Margaret, 183
Glassman, Ronald M., 210
Goldspink, Chris, 10
Goldstone, Jack A., 218
Goleman, Daniel, 51
Goody, Jack, 151
Gouldner, Alvin W., 152
Greene, Brian, 138, 216

Habermas, Jurgen, 208, 209, 213

Hebert, Paul D. N., 187
Heckathorn, Douglas D., 216,
218
Heider, Fritz, 174, 216
Hempel, Carl G., 215
Hennis, Wilhelm, 208
Hindess, Barry, 208
Hinkle, Roscoe C., Jr., 177
Hogan, James P., 152
Holland, John H., 216
Hölldobler, Bert, 187, 202
Homans, George Caspar, 188
Huff, Toby, 208
Hunt, Lynn, 53

Ibn Khaldûn, 2, 3, 12, 36, 65, 69,
70, 85, 98, 127, 137–142,
144–147, 149, 158, 162,
168–170, 188, 190, 210,
212, 216

Jastrow, Robert, 152
Jepperson, Ronald L., 216
Johnson, Barclay D., 197
Jones, Robert Alun, 52, 177, 185,
215
Jones, Susan Stedman, 181, 185

Kalberg, Strphen, 208
Kanter, James, 3
Kauffman, Stuart, 3, 6, 23, 174,
187, 216
Kellner, Douglas, 208
Keynes, Richard, 21
Klein, Richard G., 188
Knobe, Joshua, 175, 214
Kroeber, A. L., 13, 188

Leakey, Richard, 22, 217
LeBon, Gustave, 200
Lenski, Gerhard E., 146
Levine, Donald N., 208
Levi-Setti, Riccardo, 216
Levy, Marion J., Jr., 151

Lewin, Roger, 22, 23, 217
Lim, May, 188
Lindholm, Charles, 125
Lindley, David, 6
Luckmann, Thomas, 49, 177
Lukes, Steven, 177, 182, 186, 191, 198, 199, 206, 215
Luther, Martin, 131, 132, 134

Malthus, Thomas, 1, 11, 18–24, 34, 35, 83, 84, 127, 144, 162, 163, 166–169, 188, 190, 201
Mannheim, Karl, 5, 217
Marcuse, Herbert, 103, 124, 208
Marks, Stephen, 193
Martindale, Don, 208
Marwell, Gerald, 216
Marx, Karl, 11, 21, 28, 29, 46, 48, 65, 105, 110, 118, 123, 124, 127, 128, 132–135, 135–139, 144, 150, 152, 162–168, 170, 188–195, 199, 201–206, 211, 214, 218
McFarland, Daniel, 188
Mead, George Herbert, 15, 194, 207
Merton, Robert K., 13, 21, 179, 186, 188, 189, 191, 216
Metzler, Richard, 188
Miller, George A., 49
Mills, C. Wright, 124
Mommsen, Wolfgang J., 108, 110, 208
Moody, James, 188
Morowitz, Harold J., 216
Moss, Scott, 188
Murvar, Vatro, 210

Nisbet, Robert, 180, 182, 183, 185
Nozick, Robert, 208

Ogburn, William Fielding, 149

Oliver, Pamela E., 216
Orum, Anthony M., 208

Pareto, Vilfredo, 116, 143, 215, 217
Parkin, Frank, 208
Parsons, Talcott, 13, 50, 109, 124, 178, 184, 188, 200, 208
Pascal, R., 194
Pickering, W.S.F., 52
Pope, Whitney, 177, 179, 180, 215
Popper, Karl R., 69, 208, 209, 215

Rawls, Anne Warfield, 181, 182
Riedel, Johannes, 208
Ritzer, George, 184, 188, 193, 197, 208
Robertson, Roland, 216

Sample, Ian, 187
Sayer, Derek, 207, 208
Schluchter, Wolfgang, 130, 208
Schroeder, Ralph, 118, 208
Segady, Thomas W., 208
Semple, Ellen Churchill, 214
Shibutani, Tomotsu, 216
Shils, Edward, 122–124, 210
Shubin, Neil, 189, 196
Sica, Alan, 208
Siebold, David R., 10
Simmel, Georg, 49, 120, 126, 191–193, 201, 209, 211
Simon, Herbert A., 216
Skvoretz, John, 216
Smith, Adam, 18, 29, 30, 35, 70, 71, 84, 163–165
Sowell, Thomas, 148
Spencer, Herbert, 4, 27, 144, 153, 194, 195, 206, 212, 213
Stoeckle, Mary Y., 187
Swatos, William H., Jr., 210
Swidler, Ann, 208

Swift, Jonathan, 190
Tekla, Tendzin N., 180, 215
Tenbruck, Friedrich H., 208
TenHouten, Warren, 180, 191
Thomas, Dorothy Swaine, 210
Thomas, William I., 210
Thompson, Kenneth, 191
Tilly, Charles, 190, 189
Tiryakian, Edward A., 180, 185, 191
Tominaga, Ken'ichi, 208
Toynbee, Arnold J., 212
Traugott, Mark, 180, 181, 184
Treur, Jan, 187
Turner, Brian S., 179, 197
Turner, Jonathan, 177, 208

Van Frassen, Bas C., 215
Veblen, Thorstein, 20, 203, 206, 211, 215
Vilenkin, Alex, 174, 214
Voight, Benjamin F., 5

Von Bertalanffy, Ludwig, 172, 216

Wagner, David G., 216
Waldrop, M. Mitchell, 218
Wallace, Walter L., 9, 12, 29, 212
Ward, Peter D., 5, 7, 23, 218
Watt, I., 150
Weber, Max, 1, 14, 97–136, 147, 162, 174, 200, 202, 207, 209–211, 213
Weiss, Johannes, 208
Wen, Xiaoquon, 5
Wheeler, John Archibald, 218
Wiley, Norbert, 208
Wilson, Edward O., 186
Wuthnow, Robert, 208
Wrong, Dennis, 208

Zinsser, Hans, 147